Practical Pre-School

Physical Development

Keeva Austin

Contents

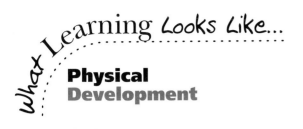

About this book

This book takes a close look at one of the six areas of learning in the curriculum guidelines across the United Kingdom - Physical Development in England, Wales and Northern Ireland, Physical Development and Movement in Scotland.

Guidance and good practice

The author explains what the area of learning consists of, what the jargon means and how it applies to the various settings in the Foundation Stage of education - children aged between three and five.

There are four different curriculum bodies across the United Kingdom - the Qualifications and Curriculum Authority (QCA) in England; the Curriculum and Assessment Authority for Wales (Awdurdod Cwricwlwm Ac Asesu Cymru); the Scottish Consultative Council on the Curriculum; and the Northern Ireland Council for the Curriculum Examinations and Assessment. Each has a different statement relating to the desired curriculum for young children. However, although there are some differences in terminology and some slight variations in emphasis, good practice in one country is still considered good practice in another. The text includes references throughout to the different systems which allows early

years practitioners to put the correct terms in their planning and for inspection purposes.

As well as giving theoretical guidance - albeit in practical terms - the book also offers suggestions for activities which can be used to deliver the curriculum requirements.

Practical activities

All these activities should be considered as merging into the normal life of the early years setting. The book stresses the importance of play and how the different areas of learning are linked. The activities are not prescriptive and should not be seen as tasks to complete. They are designed to be manageable and fun.

There are suggestions for 15 activities. Some are simple and straightforward activities which need few resources. Others are deliberately more challenging. Each can be used in some form with children at different stages of development.

The activities are planned to cover all the Physical Development Early Learning Goals (ELGs). Many of the ELGs overlap and interrelate with one another. The activities therefore often fulfil more than one ELG.

All the activities follow the same format:

❑ The learning objectives are outlined.

❑ Suggestions are made for getting started.

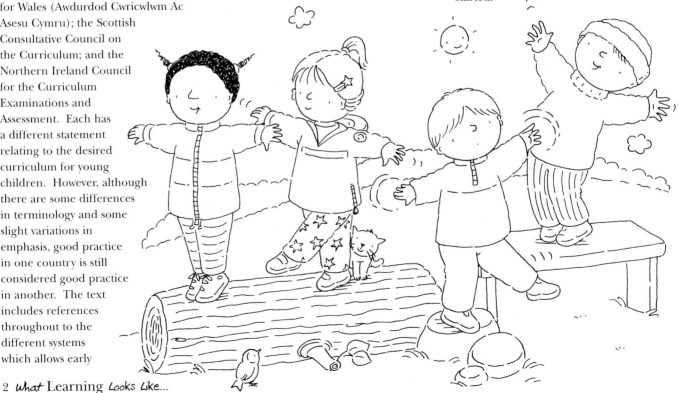

❏ The activities are then divided into stages from 1-3. (Stage 1 is the easiest and stage 3 the hardest.)

❏ Ideas for assessment are also given.

❏ Where relevant, suggestions are made for further activities and books linked to the theme. These activities are linked to the theme and can be implemented alongside the main physical activity.

The activities are staged to show progression through physical development. All children develop at different rates. Children within the Foundation Stage, move along a continuum and their progress will not necessarily be steady or uniform. We must not focus on age appropriate activities but developmentally appropriate activities. Within your group you will probably have children working at all three of the suggested activity levels.

These activities are only ideas and should not be seen as prescriptive models! You may want to adapt and change them to make them more appropriate for the group of children you are teaching.

It is also important to remember that although children do make progress within the Foundation Stage in the area of Physical Development, it is not only due to maturation but as a result of being given the time to practise, repeat and refine their physical skills.

Planning

A planning chart has been included for support and guidance but we would encourage you to adapt this readily to meet your own needs and circumstances.

There are seven books in this series, and although each book can be used by itself, they are designed to fit together so that the whole learning framework is covered.

The seven titles are:

❏ Personal, Social and Emotional Development

❏ Communication, Language and Literacy

❏ Mathematical Development

❏ Knowledge and Understanding of the World: Geography and History

❏ Knowledge and Understanding of the World: Science and Technology.

❏ Physical Development

❏ Creative Development

All of these books carry some activities based on common themes which, when used together, will give enough ideas for a cross-curricular topic over a half or even a full term.

The common themes are:

❏ Seasons

❏ Water

❏ Colour

❏ All about me

❏ People who help us

All the books together provide an outline of the learning which should be taking place in the Foundation Stage.

Assessment

Each activity includes an assessment section. Assessment involves two distinct activities:

❏ The gathering of information about the child's capabilities.

❏ Making a judgement based on this information.

Assessment should not take place in isolation. We assess to meet individual needs and ensure progress. The following tips may help your assessment to be more effective.

❏ Assessment is a continuous process. It should be systematic to ensure all children are observed on a regular basis.

❏ Assessment should always start with the child. The first steps in providing appropriate provision is by sensitively observing children to identify their learning needs.

❏ Assessment should not take place to see how much the child has learned but should take place to plan appropriately for future activities.

❏ You should be a participant in the assessment process, interacting and communicating with the child.

The main way of assessing the young child is through careful observation.

Observations should:

❏ Record both the positive and negative behaviour shown.

❏ Be long enough to make the child's behaviour meaningful.

❏ Record only what you see and not what you think you have seen or heard.

❏ Be clear - before you begin be sure you know what you want to observe.

❏ Be organised - plan ahead, otherwise it will not happen.

Physical Development

National guidelines

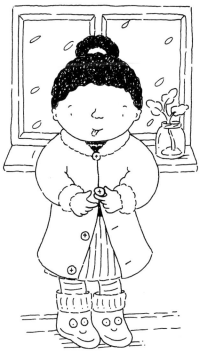

All four countries in the United Kingdom have their own document relating to the recommended curriculum for children aged from three years old to the beginning of the relevant national curriculum.

Like the previous English Desirable Learning Outcomes, the Northern Ireland (NI), Welsh and Scottish curricular guidance documents are for children in the year prior to compulsory education, in other words for children in their pre-school year.

All four documents stress that provision for children of this age is not universal and can take place in a variety of settings (primary schools, nursery units, private nursery schools, day nurseries or pre-schools). At the same time all documents recognise the importance of parents and emphasise that many of the child's most valuable experiences will continue to take place at home.

With the exception of the English document, the others stress that the key aspects or areas of learning are not discrete, separate subject areas. Children should experience them in a holistic way with learning ranging across all areas and with one area frequently re-inforcing another.

The Scottish, Welsh and Northern Ireland documents place the areas of learning firmly in context. They all stress:

❑ The importance of pre-school education and the characteristics of the pre-school child.

❑ The importance of promoting good practice and effective learning in terms of planning, observation, evaluation and record keeping.

The English Early Learning Goals

The Early Learning Goals (ELGs) are part of the English Foundation Stage which was established to define the curriculum entitlement for children from the age of three to the end of the Reception year.

The purpose of the goals is to set out what most children are reasonably expected to achieve by the end of their Reception year and provide a basis for long-term planning of the curriculum. The goals are broken down into learning activities for children at various stages of their development. These are described as stepping stones. The stepping stones should be used in planning to help the children achieve the ELG which forms the final stepping stone. Stepping stones are not age-related.

The *Curriculum Guidance for the Foundation Stage* is organised into six areas of learning: Personal, Social and Emotional Development, Communication, Language and Literacy, Mathematical Development, Knowledge and Understanding of the World, Physical Development and Creative Development.

The document attaches particular importance to Personal, Social and Emotional Development. It stresses

that this area of learning is a pre-requisite for all other areas and should be nurtured during all activities.

Physical Development

The *Curriculum Guidance* stresses the importance of using both the outdoors and indoor environment to promote gross and fine motor movements. It says that young children's physical development is inseparable from any other aspects of development because children learn through being active and interactive.

The skills and ability children should have mastered by the end of the Foundation Stage are as follows:

Early Learning Goals for movement
❑ move with confidence, imagination and in safety (ELG 1)

❑ move with control and coordination (ELG 2)

❑ travel around, under, over and through balancing and climbing equipment (ELG 3)

> For ease of reference these goals have been numbered, as indicated, so that cross-references can be made throughout the text to show where activities support work towards these goals.

Early Learning Goals for a sense of space

❑ show awareness of space, of themselves and of others (ELG 4)

Early Learning Goals for health and bodily awareness

❑ recognise the importance of keeping healthy and those things which contribute to this (ELG 5)

❑ recognise the things that happen to their bodies when they are active (ELG 6)

Early Learning Goals for using equipment

❑ use a range of small and large equipment (ELG 7)

Early Learning Goals for using tools and materials

❑ handle tools, objects and malleable materials safely and with increasing control (ELG 8)

The Northern Ireland Curricular Guidance for Pre-School Education

The NI document talks about the range of learning opportunities children should have through play and other relevant experiences. These are set out under seven headings, similar to the English and Welsh ones with the exception of Knowledge and Understanding of the World, which is divided into two:

❑ Early Experience in Science; and

❑ Technology and Knowledge and Appreciation of the Environment.

The document attaches particular importance to Personal, Social and Emotional Development as a pre-requisite for all other areas.

Physical Development

Physical Development is outlined in terms of the anticipated progress children will make, stressing that children progress at different rates. Initially physical play is described in general terms giving a description of what physical development involves: fine and large motor skills, hand-eye co-ordination, and self-confidence and social skills. It then sets out the characteristics of satisfying physical play in terms of the suitability of space, the equipment offered and the way in which it is organised and the role of the adult. It specifically mentions indoor play and offers guidance on implementation.

The document describes the skills children will be developing - physical control, mobility, awareness of space and manipulative skills. It emphasises the importance of establishing positive attitudes towards a healthy life.

It explains how other areas contribute to physical development by providing examples.

Rather than listing specific goals it gives general descriptions called 'Progress in learning' which outline the characteristics and skills most children should be demonstrating if they have received appropriate pre-school education.

Like the English document, the NI one stresses the importance of using both the outdoors and indoor environment to promote gross and fine motor movements. The key areas which need to be encouraged are:

❑ The development of awareness of self and of space.

❑ The ability to move with confidence, control, co-ordination and safely.

❑ Opportunities to use small and large equipment and tools. It gives suggestions as to the type of skills the children may be involved in when using the equipment - running, hopping, jumping and balancing.

The Welsh Desirable Outcomes for Children's Learning before Compulsory School Age

The Welsh document also divides the areas of learning into six areas, but instead of goals has Desirable Learning Outcomes (DLOs).

It stresses that the DLOs should not be seen as a self-contained check-list but

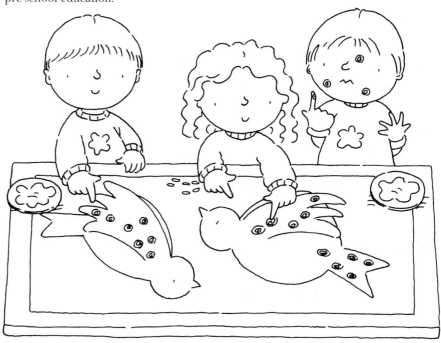

are a part of the learning activities offered to children. It recognises that the developmental continuum encompasses a wide range of ability and progress along it is not necessarily steady or uniform.

Physical Development

Like the English document, it introduces the DLOs by describing the skills children will be developing - physical control, mobility, awareness of space and manipulative skills.

It also emphasises the importance of establishing positive attitudes towards a healthy life specifically emphasising the importance of diet, rest and sleep and hygiene.

The skills and ability children should have mastered by the end of the stage are:

❏ To move confidently with increased control and co-ordination.

❏ To have an awareness of space (called spatial relationships in the Welsh document).

❏ To be able to use small and large equipment. Examples are given: bike, ball and climbing frame.

❏ To handle tools and objects with increased control (again with examples).

The Scottish Curriculum Framework

The Scottish document refers to planned learning experiences based on different key aspects of children's development and learning.

The key aspects are divided into five areas with each area described in terms of a number of features of learning. The areas are broadly the same as the English and Welsh documents. Creative Development is known as Expressive and Aesthetic Development. There is no mathematical key aspect; instead mathematical experiences are part of Knowledge and Understanding of the World.

The document attaches particular importance to Personal, Social and Emotional Development. It stresses that this area of learning is a pre-requisite for all other areas and should be nurtured during all activities.

The Scottish document is the most detailed of

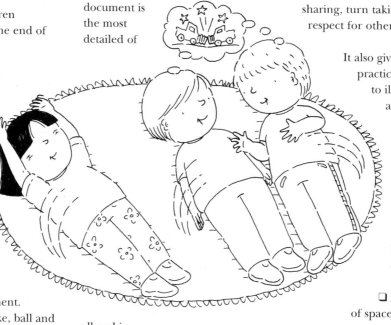

all and is different from the ELGs.

Physical Development and Movement

The curriculum framework refers to key aspects of learning of which Physical Development and Movement is one. The document emphasises that physical development and movement are closely linked with other aspects of learning and influenced by a child's

growing confidence and enjoyment of physical play; an increased ability to control their bodies and physical well-being and strength.

It stresses that children become more controlled and co-ordinated in their physical movements when they practise, experience and explore what their bodies can do.

This document emphasises the importance of enjoyment. It also describes how children should be encouraged to use their bodies to express ideas and feelings in response to music or imaginative ideas.

It sees physical play as a social activity where children develop the skills of sharing, turn taking, negotiating and respect for others.

It also gives examples from practice which are designed to illustrate how the key aspects interrelate. The examples are also given to aid planning.

It emphasises the need for indoor and outdoor play.

Physical play should develop:

❏ An awareness of space.

❏ An awareness of the importance of health and fitness.

❏ A child's skills of control and co-ordination. (The document gives examples - hands and eyes for throwing and catching or legs and arms for skipping.)

❏ The ability to handle tools and equipment.

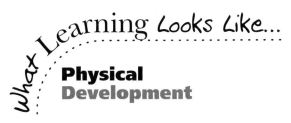
Physical Development

The area of learning explained

The early years are a time of rapid physical and mental development as young children learn to control and use their bodies and become aware of what they can do and what it is possible to do.

Movement milestones

When a baby is born his whole body moves without any co-ordination. Slowly the child is able to use parts of his body independently of each other. It is his urge to explore his immediate surroundings that motivates him to smile, reach out, roll over, crawl, shuffle, sit and eventually stand up and walk unaided. This series of movement milestones - the stages in physical development - follow the same basic sequence in all children and for most of them the milestones are natural and inevitable.

These milestones can be compared to the stepping stones in the *Curriculum Guidance*. They are not age related but children will progress through them until they reach the Early Learning Goals.

They will:

❏ Use large muscles before small ones (they roll before picking up a spoon).

❏ Control the upper part of their body before the lower half (they lift their head before they stand).

❏ Move their arms before their fingers.

❏ Make big unco-ordinated movements before small ones.

Even without help most children eventually walk, run and balance by themselves.

As the child follows this pattern and learns to move, the acquisition of greater strength, agility, co-ordination,

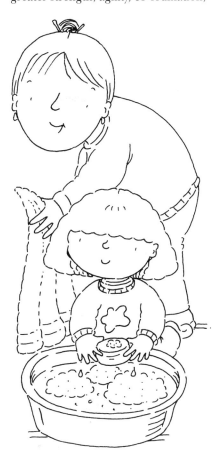

balance and control of his body mark his development. His understanding of the concepts of distance, height, and space increases.

Motor movements are divided into two kinds.

Gross motor movements

These are movements of the large muscles of the body and include such skills as climbing, rolling, twisting, curling, walking, running, skipping and balancing. Gross motor movements also include spatial relationships. This simply means that a child should know where he is in space, how he relates to objects and people around or near him. It involves the understanding of directions, for example up/down, over/under, to the right/to the left, forwards/backwards and the understanding of position, for example inside/outside, on/in, under/over, top/bottom, and high/low. (ELG 3, 4)

Fine motor movements

These are movements which involve the use of limited individual parts of the body. It usually refers to the hands and the fingers in performing precise movements and includes such skills as cutting, writing, pasting, dressing, eating and threading. The main feature of fine motor control is that it involves the child in using his eyes and his hands simultaneously - hand-eye co-ordination. (ELG 8)

By the time a child enters pre-school or nursery at three years they have mastered the rudimentary movement abilities which form the basis for further development. It is the task of the early years practitioner to make the most of each movement milestone or stepping stone as they occur, and in doing so help the child to refine and develop these movements.

The *Curriculum Guidance* helps with this by identifying examples of what children do. These examples provide snapshots of children and help to put the stepping stones into a familiar context. Likewise the *Guidance* identifies ways in which practitioners can support and consolidate a child's learning.

Extending physical play

Young children need and enjoy plenty of opportunities to repeat and refine their emerging physical skills. How can you extend outdoor play to ensure the child is challenged and makes progress whilst still having fun?

Organising the outdoor environment

The layout and organisation of the outdoor environment is just as important as the indoor one. A safe, well-planned and resourced learning environment encourages effective learning. Children will improve their coordination, control and ability to move more effectively if they can run, climb, balance, swing, slide, tumble, throw, catch and kick when they want to and are motivated and interested in doing so. The outdoor environment should be organised into defined areas. The following examples are only suggestions. Much will depend on the space and equipment available.

❑ A throwing and kicking area. (ELG 7)

❑ A free play area where the children can move as they wish, with confidence, imagination and safety. It should be a larger area than others, giving the children the opportunity to use the space appropriately. (ELG 1, 4)

❑ A movement area for toys such as bikes, trikes and cars. (ELG 7)

❑ An area for large play equipment, such as slides, swings and climbing frames, providing children with a range of items to travel around, under, over and through, balancing and climbing when appropriate. (ELG 3, 7)

❑ A changeable area where activities can be altered, developed or adult directed. (See 'Organising the equipment'.)

Organising the equipment

Organising your resources well can extend play, encouraging children to use a range of small and large equipment. (ELG 7) Separate the equipment and label it clearly, then allow free choice and free play. At other times, limit the choice to focus on one skill and avoid the outdoor play area becoming littered with items.

Some suggestions for organisation may include items for:

❑ Throwing/catching (a selection of large/small, soft/hard balls, bean bags, hoops and quoits).

❑ Kicking (balls, boxes, balloons and stones).

❑ Balancing (planks of wood, benches, logs and stepping stones).

❑ Climbing/crawling through (climbing frames, car tyres, netting, old sheets laid on the ground, large boxes, hoops, barrels and trees with low branches).

❑ Developing agility and co-ordination (logs, stepping stones, skipping ropes for skipping and for walking along when laid on the ground, cones, tyres to walk, run or cycle in/out of).

Indoors/outdoors

Most activities you provide indoors can also be offered outdoors. Put them outdoors for a change or offer them both outside and in so that each child has a real choice. Provide fine motor activities alongside the usual gross motor ones. Some of the usual fine motor activities come into their own when placed outside.

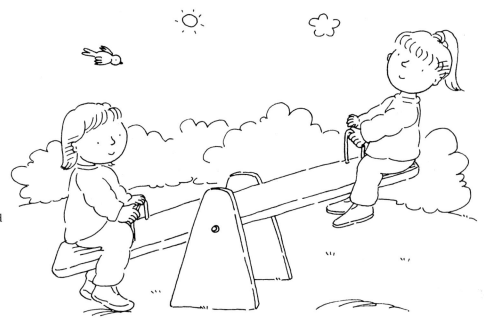

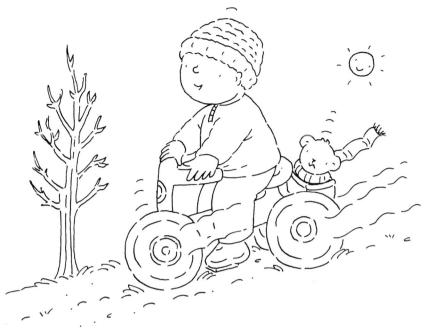

Water play can be more extravagant because spills do not matter so much. Use paddling pools for water activities during the summer and provide the children with large containers such as buckets and saucepans rather than the smaller ones usually used inside.

Painting can be more experimental, using large decorating brushes or big sheets of paper, or (if you are feeling brave!) even foot painting.

Large construction play can be more imaginative as there may be more space to work in and different materials.

Planning for Physical Development

Children enjoy energetic, physical and free play, allowing them the chance to practise, to repeat, to copy and to attempt a range of physical movements. However, although we work hard to provide the physical environment, the materials and the resources for all these activities, it is not enough just to provide them and hope children will learn. Alongside these spontaneous opportunities, planned activities need to take place. The Northern Ireland Curriculum Council (NICC) (1996) says that 'satisfying physical play takes place when: play is planned carefully, so that interest is sustained, challenge is offered and activities are balanced to provide for individual needs and abilities'.

The role of the adult is crucial in planning and providing an environment that encourages children to do things, talk about what they are doing and to think about how they can improve.

Types of physical development and skills

The ELGs are based around movement, a sense of space, health and bodily awareness and using equipment, tools and materials. In order to develop these skills we need to encourage a range of movements and activities, all of which follow a developmental sequence as suggested in the stepping stones.

Walking

The mature walking pattern is usually achieved between three and four years. You would expect children arriving at pre-school or nursery to be able to walk around carrying objects, stoop to recover objects and walk in different directions - backwards, forwards and sideways. This progresses until children are able to walk in contrasting ways, such as tiptoeing, marching, striding and creeping or at differing speeds and can switch between speeds and direction easily and effectively. Suggestions for older children may include walking together without falling over (for example, in a three-legged race) or walking along painted lines or low benches without toppling over. (ELG 1, 2, 3)

Climbing

Climbing is linked developmentally to walking. Children will attempt to go upstairs even before they can stand alone, but once able to walk they will climb the stairs in an upright position with adult support. This first attempt at climbing progresses until children are able to walk upstairs (and later downstairs) alternating their feet. Our aim during these early years should be to give the children plenty of opportunities to test and improve their climbing skills and to use small and large apparatus with increasing confidence and imagination. (ELG 1, 7)

Running

Children begin to run shortly after they learn to walk. Once they can run without falling, then their skills of control and co-ordination increase. Encourage the children to run, starting and stopping safely. Ask them to alter their walking/running pattern, for example marching in time to music or running in a circle (this demands a higher level of co-ordination!). Try running with a partner or participate in chasing games. If they are proficient, ask them to gallop. (ELG 1, 2, 4)

Jumping

This involves a good degree of co-ordination and balance. (ELG 2) You may have to show some children how to jump, not because they are physically unable to, but because they have never been asked to jump. Practice is therefore the key.

Young children enjoy jumping around with two feet together. They progress to jumping over lines or jumping off low steps. Once they can jump with increasing height, then you can encourage them to hop. Hopping is difficult, as it requires the child to regain his balance on one leg after jumping in the air. Once they can hop a few paces on one leg then encourage them to hop over a distance. The children are then ready to attempt to hop on alternate feet or play games such as hopscotch.

Skipping

This is one of the last locomotion skills to appear. It only develops as a result of practice. Children will progress from the first attempts to skip (which resemble a cross between a run and a walk!) then on to a half-stepping, half-jumping, half-skipping pattern before developing a mature skipping pattern. (ELG 2, 3)

Balancing skills

To be able to achieve the above locomotion skills effectively, children need to be able to establish and maintain their balance.

They need lots of opportunities to practise balancing. Young children can be encouraged to practise standing on tiptoes or balancing on one foot. For those children who find this easy, suggest that they try

balancing on different parts of their bodies, for example, one hand and one foot simultaneously. Much harder is the ability to balance whilst the body is moving. Encourage the children to walk along a narrow bench or ask them to walk with bean bags on their hands, backs or heads. This is an activity children seem to enjoy and with practice become skilled. (ELG, 2, 3, 7)

Manipulative skills

This involves both gross motor and fine motor movements. I concentrate here on fine motor skills. Ball skills such as throwing, catching and kicking are manipulative skills involving gross motor movements. (These are discussed as part of an activity on page 40.) This does not mean that children use either gross motor or fine motor movements. On the contrary, most activities will involve the children using these skills simultaneously.

There are few activities that do not involve hand function of some kind and children make vast progress in this area of development during their early years. For many three- to four-year-olds hand functioning will have developed enough to attempt the majority of activities you offer. It is your role to refine these skills by giving them opportunities to practise continually and improve the quality of their skills, to help them handle tools, objects, construction and malleable materials safely and with increasing control. (ELG 8)

Fine motor skills can be divided into three groups:

Malleable materials

Young children need the time to explore by touch and feel before progressing to more formal skills, including writing and drawing. Offer the children a range of messy

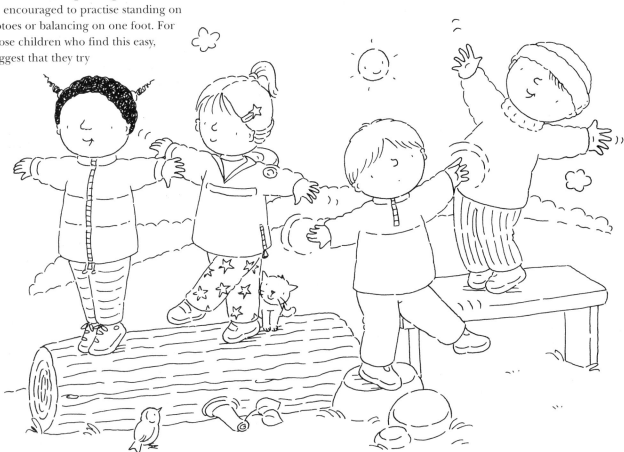

activities to stimulate their curiosity and help them learn about the properties of the materials provided.

Activities may include salt drawings, finger painting, clay or dough, cornflour slime and sand and water play. At first it is enough just to provide the experience and observe how they handle the materials. Providing appropriate equipment and sensitive adult interaction can extend their play and fine motor skills.

Construction materials

Development begins with the enjoyment of knocking over brick towers built by adults! The children progress until they are able to build their own towers and trains from bricks. As they get older and gradually become better co-ordinated (ELG 2), they will build more elaborate and interesting structures.

Provide a range of construction materials and have a good quantity of each. Different sets complement each other so allow the children to have more than one type out. As the children progress, provide them with additional materials such as gears, wheels, pulleys and other small pieces. Not only will they be developing their fine motor skills but also their scientific skills as they work out how the pieces work and fit together. They will be using mathematical skills as they estimate how many bricks they need to create a structure and discussion may follow as they plan and review what they are doing.

Hand-eye co-ordination skills

I have included under this heading skills such as completing puzzles, threading and screwing, scissors and writing and drawing skills.

All these skills require a high level of hand-eye co-ordination. Children make great progress in this area once they start nursery or pre-school. However,

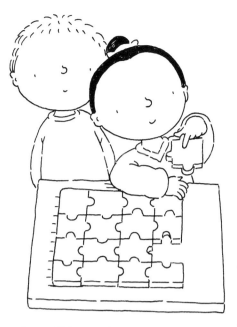

there will be a wide range of ability and this must be taken into account when providing for the children. Include simple formboards as well as interlocking puzzles. The threading tray should include a range of beads of differing sizes and shapes before you offer simple threading cards. Scissor skills move from snipping at paper to being able to cut along lines. Cutting round shapes and pictures comes much later. Concentrating for long lengths of time on these skills only leads to frustration if children are finding these skills hard (see page 13 for more on special needs).

Other fine motor skills include personal skills (dressing, feeding and toileting). Most children starting at nursery will (on the whole) be independent and need minimal support in doing up buttons, fasteners and shoe fastenings.

Games

Only the Scottish Curriculum Council (SCC) (1998) says 'In physical development and movement, children should learn to co-operate with others in physical play and games'. This document recognises that games provide children with opportunities to promote social skills. Children need to be able to share, take turns, co-operate and negotiate with each other. Introducing games also encourages spatial awareness. (ELG 4)

For the younger child this may be difficult because their level of development is still at the egocentric

stage. The games must therefore be simple and related to the child's own experiences. For example, 'What's the time Mr Wolf?', 'Simon says', and 'Follow my leader' type games would be good starting points.

As the children get older and they begin to recognise the concept of a group identity, then play becomes more co-operative and games can now include turn-taking and sharing, simple instructions and team games, for example 'Traffic lights', 'Beans', and 'Oxford and Cambridge'.

Movement and dance

Children are always expressing themselves in physical ways - stamping their foot when they're angry or jumping up and down when they're excited. Movement and dance gives children the opportunity to bring movement under conscious control and to experiment with these types of self-expression. (ELG 1) It also allows them to release feelings which may be difficult to express in other ways. In children's imagination their bodies can be and do almost anything. 'They become aware that they can use their bodies to express ideas and feelings by moving in different ways as they respond to their moods and feelings or to music or imaginative ideas' (Scottish Curriculum Council 1998).

With young children movement sessions should incorporate movements they can already do, for example ask the children to walk in different ways (not only in terms of speed and direction) but be more creative. Walk as if you were carrying a heavy load, walk as if you were very happy - fun ideas which encourage self-awareness. (ELG 4) The older the child the more you can encourage them to use their imagination, perhaps linking movement with a current theme, for example, ask them to think of an animal and move as if they were that animal.

Spatial awareness is a concept that recurs over and over in an increasingly complex way during movement/dance sessions. (ELG 4) Encourage the children to use their whole bodies to move as well as using the space around them. Encourage the use of spatial language: up/down, under/over and high/low. (ELG 3) Promote physical skills further by asking questions. You can develop their speed and strength by asking them to creep quietly and slowly like a cat, or encourage them to improve their control and co-ordination (ELG 2) by asking them to reach or jump a little higher.

Gymnastics

Gymnastics and apparatus work should never be introduced too early. It relies on controlled actions and movement and may be too difficult for the young child. Allowing children sufficient time to explore, control and co-ordinate their own bodies is more important than introducing apparatus.
(ELG 1, 2, 4)

When you do use apparatus, make sure that the

environment is large enough for the children to move comfortably and safely (ELG 1), and that the apparatus is suitable for all ages and abilities. Initially the layout should be simple and yet challenging - open to exploration and discovery by the children. Keep the layout the same for several sessions to allow the children the opportunity to refine and adapt their movements in order to build up their confidence and ensure success.

Layouts depend on equipment available, but at the simplest stage, apparatus work should always complement floor work. The aim is to give the children the opportunity to practise skills they have already learned in a different working environment. Simplicity is the key! For example, in early sessions the apparatus may be set up but the children are asked to move around the room without going on the apparatus, instead going under, over and around the equipment. Progress to using the apparatus but ask the children to think of ways of using their feet to get on, travel along and come off the apparatus. The sessions can then continue, through greater control (ELG 2) to being able to put together more and more actions that are varied

in their directions, levels and space used. (ELG 3, 7)

Looking after our bodies

This involves the two Early Learning Goals ELG 5 and 6:

❑ Recognise the importance of keeping healthy and those things which contribute to this;

❑ Recognise the things that happen to their bodies when they are active.

Keeping healthy and making the children aware of the need to look after themselves should be an integral part of the physical activity programme you provide.

Children (and adults) can be encouraged to wear appropriate clothing during physical activities. Discuss with them how they feel after exercise. Even the youngest child should have some understanding of the changes even if descriptive words are immature - sweaty, hot, panting, tired and so on. Older children may be aware of an increase in heart and pulse rates. Such a discussion should quite naturally lead to the conclusion that wearing the same clothes we arrived at school in is not appropriate! Talk about clothing worn by adults for exercise.

Keeping fit and wearing appropriate clothing, though, is not enough for a healthy lifestyle. Healthy eating needs to be promoted. Ensure the right food is available at snack or lunchtime or in the tuckshop. Adults should set an example by what they eat too!

Encourage the children to feel good about themselves and their physical skills, praise success, and ask them to repeat the things they do well. Adults should actively join in with the children's activities to show that it can be fun.

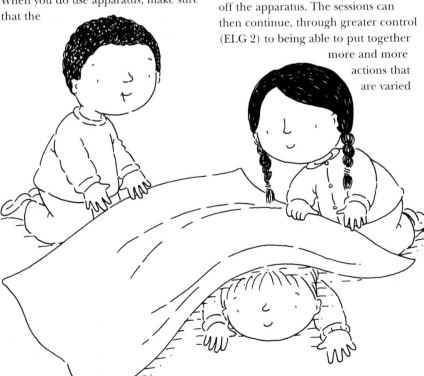

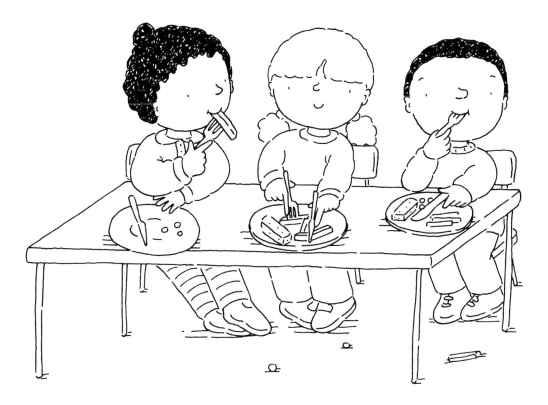

Children who find play difficult

In any group there may be a child who you would class as clumsy. He may enthusiastically join in but the harder he tries the more clumsy he becomes.

Most children will be clumsy at some stage - most new skills are learned by trial and error and repeated practice. However, the child with a real difficulty will persistently stand out. Co-ordination difficulties can affect both fine and gross motor movements. Children may have difficulty in one or both of these areas.

If there is a delay with a single activity it is not usually a cause for concern. Likewise some delays and difficulties may be due to a lack of experience. For example, if a child has never had pencils and paper at home, then he cannot be expected to know how to hold a pencil and make marks on paper. A child who is always dressed by his parent will not be able to do it for himself.

Children with real difficulties may display some or all of the following:

Fine motor

❏ Difficulties with related tasks. For example, difficulty in building bricks may mean difficulty, to, with posting shapes.

❏ Inability to undress/dress particularly with buttons, zips and shoelaces.

❏ Difficulties in throwing/catching a ball.

❏ Problems with hand-eye co-ordination, painting, drawing and spacing work on a page.

Gross motor

❏ Slow to sit up, crawl or walk.

❏ Falling or stumbling a lot.

❏ Finds balancing activities difficult.

❏ Late learning to kick a ball or ride a bike.

❏ Inability to be in the right place at the right time.

Intervention

Providing play activities appropriate to the child's developmental level can prevent minor co-ordination difficulties. (Activities to promote co-ordination include jigsaws, threading games, dot-to-dot, colouring in, dressing dolls. Body awareness activities include, drawing round hands/feet, face painting, and action songs.)

❏ Give the child time for his own unstructured play.

❏ Encourage him to practise daily routines of dressing/eating.

❏ Praise success to build up his self-esteem.

If a difficulty is more marked, then the child may need to be referred to his GP, health visitor or occupational therapist. He may have dyspraxia - an immaturity of the organisation of movement, affecting the development of motor skills. The child often has low muscle tone, a squint or instability at the shoulders or hips. Intervention will focus on teaching the child strategies to overcome his difficulty.

Links with other
areas of learning

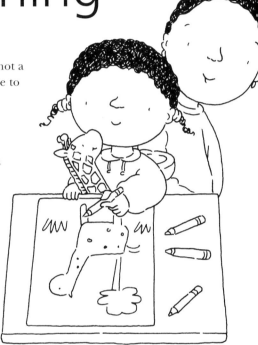

Young children's physical development is inseparable from all other aspects of development because children learn through being active. Physical Development is therefore very much linked to other areas of learning.

The topic web on the adjoining page lists some of the many activities undertaken by young children. I hope it shows that many activities which may at first be planned under another curricular heading are also fulfilling the Early Learning Goals for Physical Development. For example, the ability to hold a pencil effectively and form recognisable letters is a Communication, Language and Literacy goal, but this activity also fulfils a Physical Development goal (ELG 8): The ability to handle tools ... safely and with increasing control.

Most groups, at some time during the day, come together and talk about the weather. Although such an activity encourages the children to make comparisons between the weather on different days and perhaps record the results, this activity can also be used to discuss the types of clothes we may wear in different weather. Through this discussion the children learn how to care for themselves and keep healthy.

The web on page 15 has as its starting point the needs, interests and experiences of the children and assumes that your learning environment is well-equipped and well-organised. The types of activities suggested are ones which should be available throughout the Foundation Stage. They should be seen as an example of planned activities and not a prescriptive model - you will be able to add your own ideas. What I have attempted to do is emphasise the following points:

❑ The early years curriculum is not to be seen as separate learning areas - the ELGs are written like this to make them easy to use. In practice, learning will often overlap and link several areas of learning together and when planning it is important to try to do this.

❑ If learning is holistic and encompasses all areas then many of the examples in the web could be placed under more than one heading. For example, I have placed construction materials under Knowledge and Understanding of the World as the children compare the similarities and differences between the choice of bricks offered to them. I could have placed it under the Mathematical Development area of learning because when children are building they are having to estimate the number of bricks required and choose the necessary pieces needed to make the 3-d shapes and structures.

❑ Many activities we offer children more than adequately meet the ELGs. Rather than regarding the ELGs as prescriptive, we should see them as emphasising the good practice that takes place in many establishments.

My next two examples (see pages 16 and 17) also take the form of topic webs. This time I have tried to show how one physical activity supports, develops and meets the goals of all the other areas of learning. For example, when the children are playing outside with the bikes and cars, they will be using large pieces of equipment with confidence and co-ordination, and using space effectively. (ELG 2, 4, 7) This activity will also be reinforcing mathematical skills. The children may count the number of children on the bikes and use everyday language (in front, behind or next to) to describe their position in relation to each other.

These webs are only examples. It may be useful as a team or individually to do the same with another physical activity, for example action songs or ball skills, and see the interrelationship between the areas of learning.

Communication, Language and Literacy

❏ When drawing or writing the children are using a range of tools - pens, pencils, crayons and chalks.

❏ Children discuss how they are going to climb to the top of the climbing frame and who will get there first.

❏ In the book corner children learn to handle books and turn over pages appropriately.

❏ Drama and role-play involves movement and spatial awareness.

❏ Threading beads and pegboard skills (early reading and sequencing skills) also develop hand-eye co-ordination and fine motor control.

❏ Dot-to-dot and tracing sheets are designed to develop early reading skills, perceptual motor skills and use of tools.

❏ Many popular nursery rhymes and songs, for example 'Jack and Jill' and 'The Grand Old Duke of York', involve actions or body movements.

Mathematical Development

❏ Mathematical activities such as sorting, counting and matching develop hand-eye co-ordination and fine motor skills.

❏ In cookery through measuring, stirring, kneading and spooning the children are using manipulative skills and handling small utensils.

❏ When taking rubbings of patterns in brick work the children are developing their tactile skills.

❏ When involved in number games such as hopscotch they are having to control and co-ordinate their bodies.

Knowledge and Understanding of the World

❏ When working in the construction area they are handling construction materials safely and with increased control.

❏ Using natural materials children discover the properties of materials by handling and exploring them.

❏ Looking at a daily weather chart encourages discussion on weather change and the appropriate clothing needed to be worn (good health).

❏ Using magnifying glasses and lenses to look at mini-beasts requires hand-eye co-ordination and controlled use of small pieces of equipment.

Physical Development

Creative Development

❏ Using musical instruments to explore sound requires control and co-ordination of large and small body parts and muscles.

❏ As they create using malleable materials - clay, dough and Plasticene - children are also developing hand skills and using tools with increased control.

❏ Painting, printing, collage and junk modelling all involve the children having control over their actions as they use tools effectively.

❏ During dance, music and drama children learn how to use large muscles in a controlled way.

❏ Doll play requires good fine motor skills. For example, doing up fastenings and buttons on dolls' clothes.

Personal, Social and Emotional Development

❏ As children develop confidence in themselves, they are more eager to try new physical activities.

❏ Joining in Diwali dance celebrations promotes control of their bodies and develops spatial awareness.

❏ Dressing/undressing requires fine motor co-ordination.

❏ Children need to follow the safety rules when playing on large equipment.

❏ Children express their thoughts and feelings when painting or drawing. Both require the use of small tools.

❏ Caring for and feeding class pets requires careful handling of the animals; it also helps the children realise the importance of good hygiene.

Physical Development

Communication, Language and Literacy

❏ The children discuss what they are building with the sand using appropriate language and vocabulary.

❏ The children use the sand tray to create and draw patterns and letters in the sand using a variety of tools.

❏ Collaborative and exploratory sand play develops imagination.

❏ The children refine their listening skills when being quiet to hear the sand trickling through the funnel or sand wheel.

Mathematical Development

❏ As they build, they compare and order without measuring.

❏ Children have to estimate how much sand they need to fill containers and which holds the most.

❏ The children count the number of children at the sand tray - are there too many?

❏ They use appropriate language, for example, 'more' or 'less', 'heavier' or 'lighter' as they are building.

Personal, Social and Emotional Development

❏ Sand is a sensuous material and children can derive comfort and relaxation from handling it.

❏ Sand allows the children to create and destroy in a safe and acceptable way.

❏ Children have to learn to take turns and share the sand tray equipment.

❏ There is an agreed set of values - no throwing sand or knocking down something another child has built.

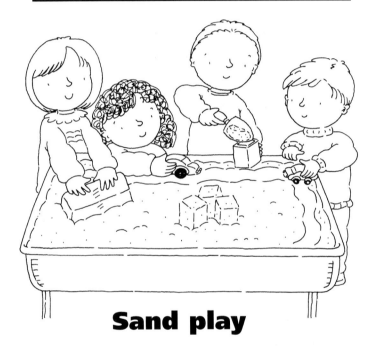

Sand play

Knowledge and Understanding of the World

❏ Playing in the sand involves using the senses to observe and investigate.

❏ The children ask questions about what they are doing. Is wet or dry sand better for pouring?

❏ Through discussion they find similarities and differences between wet and dry sand.

❏ Sand play gives them the opportunity to combine materials together, for example, water and sand - how does the sand change?

Physical Development

❏ The children handle a variety of tools and pieces of small equipment - buckets, spades, rakes and jelly moulds. As they do so they increase their control and co-ordination.

❏ Sand is a malleable material they are learning to use safely and with increasing control.

Creative Development

❏ The sand tray is used imaginatively to create whatever the children want - a building site, a beach, the zoo; the sand can be used to make cakes.

Personal, Social and Emotional Development

❏ In outdoor play the children have to learn to play in a group, to share the toys appropriately and to take turns.

❏ Using the bikes helps the children gain confidence and gives them opportunities to attempt physical challenges at their own pace.

❏ To ensure safety the children have to follow outdoor rules, for example no riding into other children.

Communication, Language and Literacy

❏ The children extend their vocabulary as they use words correctly to describe movement, direction and position. For example, forward, fast, slow, behind.

❏ They learn to listen as the adult or friend gives instructions.

❏ They use language to negotiate with each other about who is next on the bikes and which bike they will go on.

❏ The children use their developing writing skills to draw or paint a roadway on the ground.

Creative Development

❏ The children make imaginary journeys - going to the seaside, or role-play real life situations - buying petrol from the garage.

❏ They make appropriate car/bike sounds as they travel around.

❏ They are exploring space as they travel around the playground.

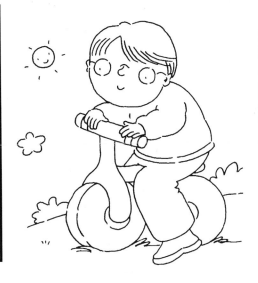

Mathematical Development

❏ Children develop understanding of one-to-one correspondence - are there enough bikes/cars for every child?

❏ Children are counting and comparing - they count how many children are on the bikes or cars. Which is the most popular?

❏ As they are cycling around they use everyday language to describe position - next to, in front of, behind. In doing so their spatial awareness develops.

Using the bikes and cars outdoors

Physical Development

❏ The children are using a range of small and large equipment.

❏ When using the bikes/cars, children are beginning to judge speed and distance.

❏ Travelling around the playground children develop an awareness of space.

❏ Practice on the bikes/cars develops their control and co-ordination.

❏ Role-play, for example taking the car to the garage, encourages use of their imaginations.

Knowledge and Understanding of the World

❏ Together the children ask questions and try to work out why certain bikes move more quickly/slowly than others.

❏ Physical play contributes to the scientific understanding of forces, pulling/pushing, stopping/starting and swerving.

❏ Playing with cars/bikes helps their understanding of road safety.

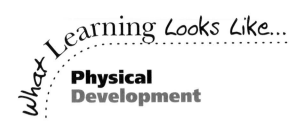

The importance of play

When an adult says to a child 'Go and play' they mean, for example, throw a ball, pretend to be a doctor, mould a Plasticene man or paint a picture. It is difficult to see what these activities have in common.

However, it appears as if all these activities are spontaneous, active and pleasurable. Play does not neccesarily depend on an adult always taking the lead. Children want to explore and learn from the world around them. Play is sometimes seen as trivial and frivolous, designed to amuse the child. But there is much more to it than that. Play is a significant activity. Purposeful play features strongly in good early years education.

Through play children are:

❏ Motivated to learn.

❏ Developing a sense of enquiry.

❏ Developing and consolidating skills.

❏ Communicating and co-operating.

❏ Playing out real-life situations in a safety.

❏ Problem-solving.

❏ Investigating and exploring the environment.

❏ Able to take risks in a secure environment.

❏ Active and absorbed.

❏ Allowed to be self-motivated and independent in their learning.

❏ Able to make choices.

❏ Provided with access to the curriculum.

The role of the adult

Play should be both structured (planned) and unstructured. Unstructured play or spontaneous play is child initiated and without the constraints of pre-determined objectives. However, just providing the opportunities and materials for children to play with is not enough. The role of the adult is important. Unless there is active teacher involvement (structured play), then the child's experiences can remain always a matter of enjoyment, satisfying immediate interests but often becoming repetitive and lacking progression. The role of the adult is therefore:

❏ To call attention to the environment and the activities by asking questions - open-ended questions which encourage them to think and therefore increase their understanding and improve language competencies. For example, 'Let's find out shall we?' or 'How do you think we could . . ?' Such interactions need to be carefully planned for. Staff have to act as a resource bank, model, guide and supporter. They are there to underpin and reinforce the planned activities.

❏ To encourage children to be active learners.

❏ To ensure the learning environment is responding to each child's needs for something familiar, something new and challenging and something which enables the child to pursue a current interest.

❏ To plan the activities but not to be so rigid as to allow spontaneous opportunities to go by. For example, if a child arrives at school with a postcard from America, give them the opportunity to show it to the group. Have any of the other children received a postcard? Where from? Perhaps get out maps of Great Britain and the world. Together find the countries on the map.

❏ To join in the play at the child's level and be willing to take turns.

❏ To show the child new ways of playing with familiar toys or activities. To bring new possibilities to an existing situation, yet not insisting the child copies you!

❏ To introduce the language of movement to children alongside their actions. Children will use new words such as 'slither' or 'gallop' if they are encouraged to. Understanding of words such as 'follow', 'lead' or 'copy' will become clearer to a child when they are associated with actions.

Structured play, then, enables the children to gain maximum learning with maximum enjoyment. It is achieved when the activities the children are involved in start with the child, their needs and interests. The activities should relate to several aspects of learning at any one time and should be well-planned including good use of all staff. Both structured and unstructured play may be appropriate at times during the week, but you need to be aware that they lead to different outcomes.

Promoting physical development through play

Physical development is perhaps one area of learning where you can immediately see a link with play. When you see a child riding a bike or kicking a ball you would say they were playing, and so often we tell children to go and play outside. It is perhaps easy, therefore, to recognise when play is supporting this area of learning. However, if we are to promote physical development more effectively through play, then it may be useful to recognise the different types of play and the skills that are developed through each.

Energetic play

Through energetic play, children are learning about what their bodies can do. Energetic play gives them the opportunity to practise new physical skills to help their developing bodies mature and become more versatile. Energetic play includes such activities as running, skipping, climbing and jumping. An essential feature of energetic play is that it often involves the whole body. Through energetic play the children are exercising the body (ELG 5), learning how to control and co-ordinate their actions (ELG 2) and move safely through space (ELG 4).

Experimental play

Children are naturally inquisitive. They want to know how things work and why. This type of play encourages them to handle tools, objects, construction and malleable materials safely and with increasing control. (ELG 8) For example, through experimenting they learn that wet and dry sand have different properties, but they also develop good hand skills by digging and building with the sand. In the water tray they need good hand-eye

co-ordination to tip and pour the water from one container to another.

Playing with large outdoor blocks allows construction on a larger scale, encouraging them to use large equipment appropriately. (ELG 3, 7)

Creative play

Children of any age love to create things and within the Foundation Stage children will be involved in a variety of creative activities. They will be painting, printing, drawing, making collages, working with dough and clay. Creative play also includes dance, drama and imaginative activities (ELG 1, 4). The Scottish Curriculum Framework document emphasises the need for children to have these opportunities to use their bodies to express ideas and feelings, as they respond to mood, music and imaginative ideas.

Through this type of play the children gain practice not only at handling tools and objects (ELG 8) but also develop more control over what they can do with their bodies with an emphasis on increasing hand skills.

Skilful play

By skilful play I mean all those games and activities which require the skilful and controlled use of the hand and eye. For example, building a tower out of bricks, completing a puzzle, playing table tennis or constructing a model. This type of play is not only important for developing such activities but also because skilful play enables a child to be more independent. Skills such as doing up buttons or feeding would come under this play heading and all involve control and co-ordination of hand and eye. As the child handles materials skilfully he is also learning about weight, shape, size, length, number, colour and sound.

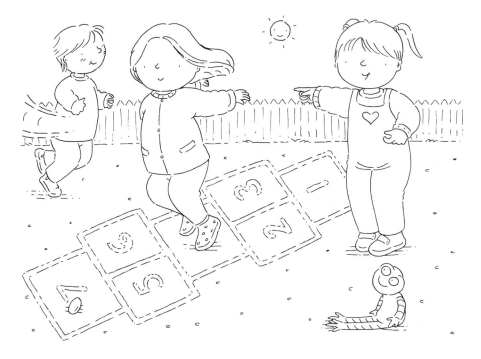

Playing with dough

Dough play is an activity that young children are offered on a regular basis. If, however, children are offered a familiar activity too frequently, there is a tendency for their play to become repetitive and lack direction. I hope that these activities provide some fresh ideas and at the same time enhance the children's learning.

Learning objectives

❑ To develop the children's exploratory skills.

❑ To enjoy using the dough.

❑ To handle tools, objects and malleable materials safely and with increasing control. (ELG 8)

Dough play gives children the opportunity to 'handle tools, objects and malleable materials safely and with increasing control' (ELG 8). The Scottish curriculum document also stresses that dough play is important for developing children's skills in using different materials (dough play being one example). It says that using the dough and the tools with it leads to increased control of fine movements of the fingers and hands. However, dough play is important for other reasons. It develops and exercises the muscles in the hands and arms. It gives the children the opportunity to create and express their ideas and feelings in a safe way. Through dough play children can create and destroy in an acceptable way. Children can also feel secure as

there is no pressure to succeed and they can easily make a new start. Manipulative and mathematical skills such as measuring, weighing, stirring, spooning and kneading are developed when the children make uncooked dough for themselves. Through dough play the children have the opportunity to see what materials feel like and how they behave.

Organisation

Dough play should be done in small groups on smooth tables. (Try working on cling-film occasionally - the dough peels off really well!) Use plastic sheeting on the tables to give the children sufficient work space -

wooden boards tends to limit their working space. Allow them time to use the materials - if children are continually waiting to join the table then introduce two dough tables!

Getting started

Using dough is primarily a sensuous activity, with children taking pleasure in the tactile experience. Initially the children should be allowed to do what they want with it. Dough offers the child the opportunity to use a material which can be changed in shape. It can be flattened, rolled, squeezed, lumped together or taken apart, yet the original quantity remains the same.

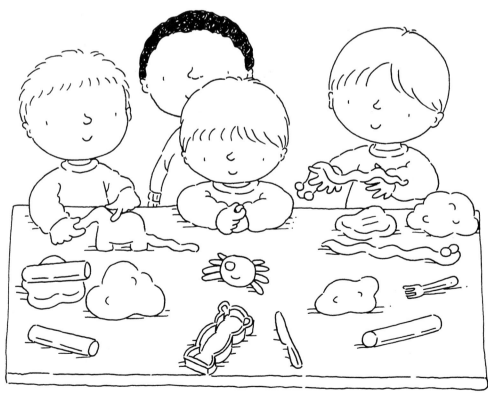

This exploration and its importance cannot be underestimated. Although children may develop useful skills such as hand control, co-ordination and the ability to use tools effectively to create complex shapes and objects from dough or clay, the stage of exploration may be returned to time and time again throughout all three stages and should not be discouraged.

Children need the opportunity and freedom to explore and use the materials without the limitations of adult ideas. However, intervention may be required to:

❏ Show children how to use certain tools;

❏ Extend their skills/ideas by working alongside a child;

❏ Motivate a child through praise and encouragement.

Exploring the material (Stage 1)

The first stage will focus on giving children the opportunity to explore the material, encouraging them to develop hand-eye coordination. At this stage the children need time to find out what the material is and what it can do. All they need is the dough itself without any utensils. Most children are happy just to handle it - squeezing, pinching, patting and holding the dough without trying to make anything.

When you feel they are ready, ask them to describe the dough - is it soft, warm, pliable, smooth or sticky? If their interest starts to wane, ask them to tell you how many things they can do with the dough and their hands - can they roll it? (Some children will have worked out how to do this for themselves, others will need to be shown.) Can they make a sausage or a ball?

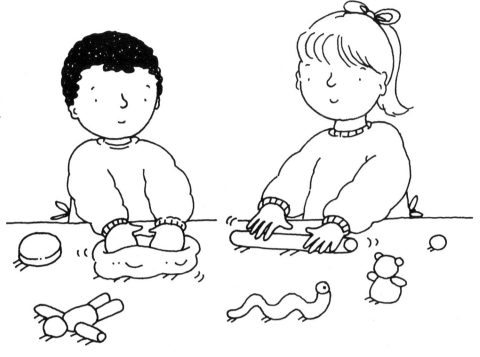

Introduce tools (Stage 2)

Stage 2 introduces tools - rolling pins, knives, spoons, lollipop sticks, forks and pastry cutters at first. At a later stage you can add other utensils - scissors, spatulas, moulds and dough machines. Remember that using tools such as a rolling pin or a cutter requires careful control and hand-eye co-ordination (ELG 2) and spatial awareness, for example, when the child is placing the cutter onto the dough.

Do not underestimate the skill involved and show the children how to use various tools if necessary. If they are not shown at this early stage they will be reluctant to return to the activity. Another important aspect of this stage of development is to encourage understanding of the importance of safety. Show them how to handle the tools in a safe way before progressing to explaining how and where the equipment is stored to ensure safety.

Children are usually happy to continue to explore the dough using the tools rather than their hands. Many children

will soon realise that as they use the tools they are creating patterns on the dough. If they do, provide them with other objects which will make different patterns (Lego, Sticklebricks, cotton reels, pencil tops, fir cones). Another time give them a selection of odds and ends (pebbles, buttons, drinking

Stages in dough play
Enjoys playing with dough
Rolls out dough using hands
Rolls out sausages
Rolls out dough using rolling pin
Able to mould shapes (circle, ball) using hands
Uses cutters to make objects
Able to cut freehand using scissors or knives to make shapes
Makes a person or other object from dough
Manipulates materials to achieve a planned effect

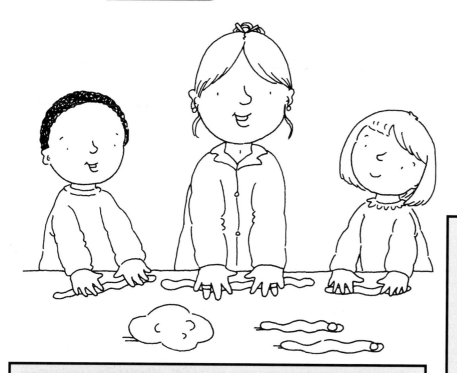

Making a necklace

❏ **Roll out the dough into sausages.**

❏ **Cut the sausages into smaller pieces (approximately 1-inch pieces).**

❏ **Make a hole through the centre of each piece using a knitting needle or similar.**

Bake the pieces for 20 minutes (Gas Mark 4/180°C).

Once cooked and cool, paint each piece in bright colours.

Thread the beads onto string to finish the necklace.

Dough recipes

Uncooked dough (salt dough)

300g plain flour

300g salt

1 tbsp oil

200ml water

Mix all the ingredients in a large bowl. The dough should feel pliable - add more liquid if necessary. Turn out onto a floured surface and knead well until very smooth and elastic. Roll or mould as required and bake in a low oven until hard.

Cooked dough

200g plain flour

100g salt

1 tbsp oil

300ml water

2 tsps cream of tartar

Few drops of food colouring

Put flour, salt, cream of tartar and oil in saucepan. Add food colouring to water. Add liquid gradually to ingredients in saucepan and mix well to get rid of any lumps. Put pan over medium/low heat and cook, stirring constantly. This is quite hard! The mixture will thicken suddenly. Stir until dough is very thick and coming away from sides of pan. Remove dough from pan and allow to cool. Once cool it can be kneaded as salt dough.

Keep in a sealed airtight container.

Dough can be cooked or uncooked. You can also alter the dough in other ways for a change:

❏ Add self-raising flour instead of plain flour to make it very stretchy.

❏ Add colour to the dough - add colouring when making it or, for a marbled effect, let the children add colour after it's been made by putting a small amount in the middle of their piece of dough and kneading it.

❏ Add smells at the cooking stage, for example, lemon juice or peppermint.

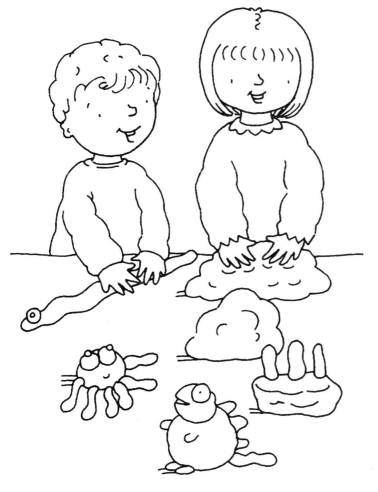

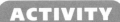

straws, sequins, bottle caps and shells). Suggest they make a dough collage using the materials. If salt dough is used for this activity then let their creations dry out before varnishing or painting them. In this way, as children move through the stepping stones, they begin to realise that using tools can effect a change in the dough.

Using dough is a good way of introducing early scissors skills. Once children have mastered the basic open/closed sequence required to cut, the children will find snipping at dough is much easier than paper and ensures success.

Making models (Stage 3)

At stage 3 children will be beginning to create their own models, manipulating the dough to achieve a planned effect. They will need the earlier skills of rolling the dough out or into sausages, snipping the dough into smaller pieces and flattening the dough. However, they may need to be shown how to:

❑ Secure two pieces of dough together - dip a finger in water and wet both surfaces or scratch the surfaces with fork.

❑ Make a hole in the dough using a cocktail stick or pencil.

❑ Roll out balls - taking a small piece of dough and making a rough ball shape before placing it in the palm of one hand and using the other hand to gently roll it out.

Older children sometimes like to make a specific item with the dough, so I have included one example, making a necklace. Use salt dough for this activity. The children can either work with an adult showing them what to do, or provide simple instruction cards.

Some children prefer to continue to work on their own without adults constantly saying, 'Why don't you make.....?' Instead, take the lead from the child and encourage and support them in their own project.

Book

You and Your Child - Playdough Ray Gibson/Jenny Tyler (Usborne).

Assessment

This will follow the progression outlined in the box on page 21. It focuses on observing children's enjoyment of dough play.

Observe if the child can:

❑ Roll out the dough using their hands or a rolling pin.

❑ Roll out the dough to make sausages, balls, flattened shapes.

❑ Use utensils and tools appropriately - cutters, scissors, knives, forks, dough machines and moulds.

❑ Use the dough to make a person or other recognisable object.

Dough play is also a very social activity and may be a good opportunity for staff to observe the children's abilities at communicating and interacting with each other as well as observing how well they are able to share and take turns with the resources provided.

Other activities

❑ Introduce clay (clay is harder to use and more difficult to work than dough) and compare the two materials. (Knowledge and Understanding of the World)

❑ Make Christmas/Diwali decorations. (Creative Development/Personal, Social and Emotional Development)

❑ Let children design their own pattern templates and transfer the design to dough. (Creative Development)

❑ Make bread dough. (Maths)

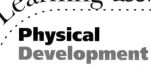
Movement patterns

Patterns is a popular theme to follow as it covers many of the areas of the curriculum, including Mathematical Development, Creative Development and Knowledge and Understanding of the World. But it can also be used in Physical Development.

Children need to have a good grasp of what is meant by pattern so you will need to put these activities in context by doing other work on patterns first.

Learning objectives

These may differ depending on your starting point. However, I have taken the following as my learning objectives:

❑ To copy, continue or create their own patterns through a variety of activities.

❑ To use fine motor skills or gross motor skills to achieve the above.

❑ To follow instructions when creating movement patterns.

These objectives will also help the children fulfil the ELGs for movement which cover 'move with control and co-ordination' and 'with confidence, imagination and in safety' (ELG 1, 2). For older children it will also include using 'a range of large and small equipment' (ELG 7).

Copying and repeating patterns

At stage 1 the activities focus on simple copying and turn taking, which encourages them to manage their own bodies and create intended

movements. Management of the children may be easier at this stage in a small group, giving the children more opportunity to share ideas and develop their thoughts.

Start with the children sitting in a circle. Begin by going round the circle, saying each child's name in turn. Create a pattern by alternating the level of your voice - first name said loudly, the second name quietly, the third name loudly, and so on round the circle. Repeat the game again but this time alter the speed at which the names are said - quickly then slowly, encouraging the children to combine and repeat a range of movements.

Once the children see the emerging pattern, introduce simple patterns through body movements. Start with the children imitating your body patterns. For example, touch head, clap hands, touch head, clap hands and so on. When they are copying you consistently see if they can continue or repeat a pattern round the group. Take a pattern already imitated. This time the first child touches his head, the second child claps his hand, the third child touches his head, and so on round the group.

At this stage you are only expecting the children to recognise body parts and such an activity should therefore be accessible to even the youngest of children. Extend the activity and introduce simple action and directional words. At this stage these would include:

Action words - stand, sit and kneel.

Directional words - forwards and backwards.

Use the idea of copying and repeating patterns outlined above to include these words. For example, sit, stand, sit, and stand. Try a harder pattern: stand, move forwards, and sit. Once they are easily copying these more difficult movement patterns you could introduce activities from stage 2.

Greater control and co-ordination

For children who are ready to move through the stepping stones, begin again in small groups. This time not only are you making the patterns more difficult in terms of the number of patterns to be repeated - three or four - but you are increasing the difficulty of the action and directional words you are expecting the children to understand.

Introduce the following action words: jump, bend, lift and kick and introduce sideways as the directional word. Repeat as for stage 1 using these words.

For example, ask the children to copy the following patterns:

Jump, bend your knees, lift your arm, jump, bend your knees, and lift your arm.

Stand, jump sideways, sit, stand, jump sideways, and sit.

These activities will not only produce increasingly complex patterns but will also encourage greater control and co-ordination (ELG 2) and movements through space (ELG 4).

Creating and recording patterns

For children working at the later stepping stones, stage 3 continues by building on stages 1 and 2. The children will by now be familiar with copying patterns and should be ready to create their own. Start by encouraging them to initiate new combinations of movement and gesture. Then encourage them to work in pairs to do this. Their pattern creations can later be shown to the rest of the group. Ask the children how they might record their patterns, so others can repeat them. (The group may have to devise a recording system, which is understood by all.) Similarly, you could have ready prepared movement cards. Can the children copy a pattern when in a pictorial form?

Further progression can include more complex action words - balancing, hopping and turning; and directional words - right and left. These action and directional words are difficult concepts to grasp. If a child is having difficulty, revert back to an earlier stage.

If, however, the children become adept at producing their own patterns then small equipment or the use of musical instruments could be introduced.

Books

The Doorbell Rang P Hutchins (Bodley Head).

The Patchwork Quilt J Pinkney/ V Flournoy (Bodley Head).

Pompaleerie Jig D Thompson/ K Baxter (Arnold Wheaton).

Other activities

❑ In the mathematics or fine motor area, activities could include creating patterns using the pegs/pegboards or beads.

❑ In the building area have a selection of bricks and construction kits.

❑ In the writing area provide materials to encourage early writing patterns.

❑ In the sand area provide items which the children can use to make patterns. For example, sand combs, rakes, sticks, potato mashers, and Lego bricks.

❑ In the painting area provide potatoes or other objects which the children can use for printing.

Assessment

When assessing the children you are not so much looking at their ability to create patterns (although being able to move with confidence and imagination may include pattern work), but at their ability to move with control and co-ordination.

You can assess this by observing at what level the children are at along the physical continuum. Stage 1 is the easier level and stage 3 the hardest. Remember, though, physical development isn't always due to maturation but due to experience and practice. To get an accurate assessment, therefore, the children may need to be observed over a period of time.

Stage 1
Action words: stand, sit and kneel.

Directional words: forwards, backwards.

Stage 2
Action words: jump, bend, lift and kick.

Directional words: sideways.

Stage 3
Action words: balance, hop and step.

Directional words: right, left.

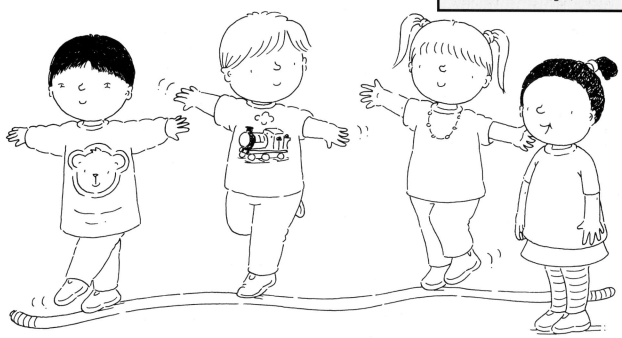

I can be a car!

These activities are designed to encourage children to use their imagination to move in different ways. You need a theme to focus ideas and transport is a good one. All children will be able to offer some experience and understanding which they can bring and share with their group and which can be used by staff to build and plan learning activities.

It is a particularly appropriate theme to use for a movement session as transport helps us move efficiently from one place to another. You may want to include these ideas as part of an overall theme on Transport. If not you'll still need to have an initial discussion about how vehicles move to put the activities in context.

Learning objectives

❑ To use music and imagination to inspire movement.

❑ To work as part of a group when necessary.

In achieving these objectives the children will also have to show an awareness of space, of themselves and others, move with control and co-ordination and be able to travel around, under and over. (ELG 2, 3, 4)

Getting started

A good starting point for young children is to ask, 'Who has a car at home?' (Include the wider family for children who may not have a car.) Discuss with them why they have a car and when they use their car. Where do they go? Using a collection of toy

vehicles (cars, trains, boats, lorries, buses and aeroplanes) widen the discussion. As the children handle, discuss and name the vehicles they can begin to classify them into groups - road transport, water transport, rail/air transport. What are the similarities/differences between these modes of transport? Encourage the children to think about how these vehicles move and the sounds they make - can the children give examples?

For older children the starting point may be the same but the discussion should be more in-depth. Ask them to think about the journeys they make. Rather than use the car could they walk or go by bus? If not, why not? Such a discussion will help them to think about travel in terms of distance, speed and time.

Move the discussion on and encourage them to begin to think of transport and travel in terms of body movements. How would they move, for example, if they were pretending to be a fast car? What parts of their bodies could they move and how?

Physical activities can become separated from other areas of the curriculum. They should not be isolated from other activities taking place. To achieve this continuity, plan the environment to reinforce physical activities. Set up a transport corner. Display appropriate books and posters (see book list) which can be used for lively discussion. Move any transport resources you may have into this corner as well - the train sets, cars and garages, Playmobil airport or harbour.

(Have you ever given the children the opportunity to have all these items out together?) Encourage the children to use them imaginatively, using their fine motor skills as they do so. Encourage the children to work out how to make the cars go faster - what happens when they use ramps or give the car a push? How do the trains link together as they go round the track?

The role of the adult is important, not only to observe and record some of their answers but to retain these records and incorporate them into the movement sessions. If the children are moving like cars in the hall, how will you recognise that it is a car? What parts of their body will they move? Can they form a line of cars and move together down a road? If the children have to recall how the cars move on the classroom roads then this may well lead to more controlled and co-ordinated movements in the hall. (ELG 2, 7)

Rhymes and action songs

With children working within the early stepping stones, confine movement to a limited range of body actions. Make the most of the many early rhymes and action songs on this theme, for example, 'I ride my little bicycle', 'Row, row, row your boat' and 'Aeroplanes, aeroplanes up in the sky' (see pages 28-29).

Songs lend themselves to larger groups with the children sitting in a circle. Once the songs and routines are familiar, then a larger space can be used with the children moving around the room more freely and

I ride my little bicycle

I ride my little bicycle,
I bought it from the shops,
And when I see a big red light,
I know it's time to stop.

I ride my little bicycle,
Not too fast or slow,
And when I see a big green light,
I know it's time to go.

The children sit in a circle.
When the song begins, ask them to
lie back on the floor with their legs
bent, then start bending and
straightening their legs as if they
are riding a bike. They have to
stop/start at the appropriate point.

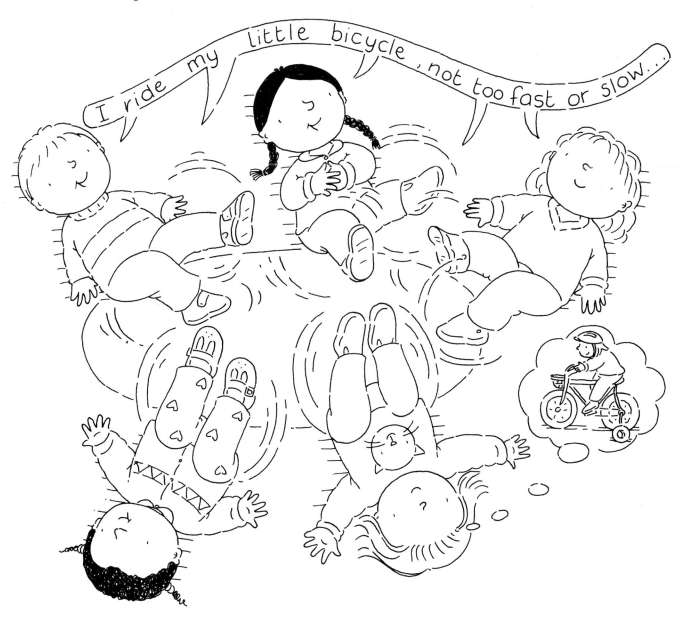

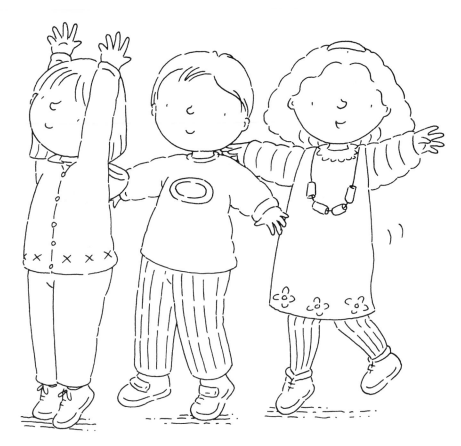

spontaneously within the available space. Another important skill to develop at this stage is the ability to stop when asked - this can often take lots of practice!

As the children's spatial awareness increases then you can suggest more elaborate movements.

Driving in your car

As children progress through the stepping stones, ask them to think of a vehicle, for example a car. Encourage them to use their imagination - taking hold of the steering wheel, looking into the mirror, accelerating and moving off. You may need to introduce some new words into your discussions beforehand to make sure the children understand the language you are using.

Begin by practising start and stop sequences, encouraging them to use space effectively (ELG 3). When the children are ready, introduce different speeds, moving very slowly-slowly-quickly-very quickly and stopping suddenly. Create an imaginary journey along a straight road then a twisting road. Small equipment (ELG 7) such as cones or tyres can be introduced at this stage. When they are confident, encourage them to adjust their speed or change direction to avoid obstacles. Older or more able children can begin to follow directions called out by the adult. For example, stop and turn right, move forwards and then reverse. (ELG 1, 2)

Introduce traffic lights. Talk about what each colour light means and the sequence in which they change from one colour to another (red - stop, amber - get ready, green - go, amber - slow down, red - stop). As the children progress, suggest that they create a complete road layout (similar to an obstacle course). Ask them to plan it out for themselves using small and large equipment (ELG 7) to create

roundabouts, road junctions and zebra crossings for example. You may like to encourage much older children to create a road layout in the classroom using the miniature play sets and then transfer their ideas into the large outdoor or indoor physical play space. Such an activity will develop directional skills, for example moving round in a circle, rotating and moving between obstacles or, if more than one child is using the road layout, ask them, 'Who is behind you?', 'Who is opposite you?' This demands good control and use of space. (ELG 2, 4)

Group work

Group work involves maturity and will probably be for older children, who can move on from cars to include different forms of transport. They can begin to work in pairs or as a whole group on more elaborate movement sequences. Perhaps working as a whole group they can pretend to be a train. Together they will need to decide how to move rhythmically. Can they form carriages and travel together without falling over and colliding? (Particularly difficult if the train is moving fast!)

In pairs can they begin to produce a sequence of movements to show how

certain vehicles move? Introduce more obscure vehicles such as tractors and trailers, bulldozers or a steamroller. Discussion will not only centre on the movement but also the mechanisms and different parts of the vehicle that are moving simultaneously. What parts of their bodies can they use to show this? Emphasise the need for movements which show strength, exaggeration and repetition. Encourage them to use their voices to make appropriate sounds as they move.

Assessment

Assessment of the children's movements can focus on their ability to move in certain ways:

❏ Direction/position - forwards, backwards, under, behind, in front of, sideways, between, left and right.

❏ Speed - slowly, quickly.

❏ Alongside this you can observe the child's ability to control and co-ordinate movements, use space effectively and move imaginatively.

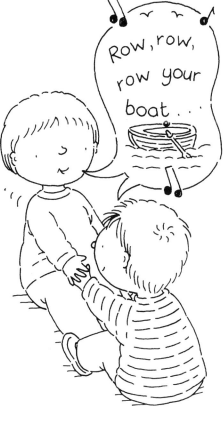

Row, row, row your boat

Row, row, row your boat,
Gently down the stream,
Merrily, merrily, merrily, merrily,
Life is but a dream.

Row, row, row your boat,
Gently down the stream,
And if you see a crocodile,
Don't forget to scream!

The children work in pairs, facing one another with their legs outstretched in front of them. They take hold of each others' hands and rock gently back and forth.

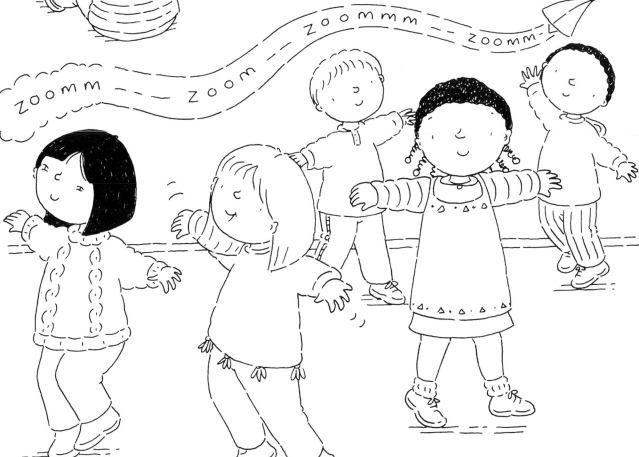

Aeroplanes, aeroplanes up in the sky

Aeroplanes, aeroplanes, up in the sky,
Aeroplanes ready to fly,
Now they're beginning to buzz and to hum,
Engines are ready so come along, come.
Now they are flying so high in the sky,
Faster and faster and ever so high.

The children find a space. They have both arms stretched out either side of their body and move their arms up and down. As the aeroplane moves faster they also rock their bodies from side to side.

Wrapping presents and parcels

In this activity, the children start with a challenge - being asked to wrap up a present. The role of the adult in the first instance is to provide a range of materials and resources to help them achieve this.

Giving the children regular access to a range of materials develops their capacity for problem-solving and lateral thinking. It develops their ability to use tools (scissors, glue, pencils) appropriately and with increasing control. It allows the children important practice at handling and controlling small items. Mathematical understanding is developed through sorting and matching shapes and colours and comparing size and texture.

The activity will also encourage them to make new discoveries, stimulate their curiosity and give them the opportunity to learn about the properties of the materials provided.

Learning objectives

❑ For the children to wrap a present unaided.

❑ To achieve this they will be developing their abilities 'to handle tools, objects, construction and malleable materials safely and with increased control'. (ELG 8)

It is the process and not the outcome, which is the focus of the activity.

Getting started

All the children (with the exception of a small minority) will have given or received a present at some time. Initial discussions may focus on the occasion when the gift was given or received.

Within most groups there will be a rich diversity of backgrounds, cultures and religions. Incorporate this into the discussion. Compile a list of all the examples the children give to each other - birthdays, Christmas, Diwali, baptism, birth of a baby, Eid, Hanukkah, Mother's Day. An appropriate book to read at this point is *A Present for Mum* by Joan Solomon (Hamish Hamilton).

If someone in the group has recently received presents, use their experience and encourage them to share with the rest of the group - why did they receive presents? What did they get and from whom?

Older children may want to think about not only when gifts are given but why? (To mark a special event, to say thank-you, to show appreciation or love and to celebrate). How do they feel when they receive or give a present?

Using a selection of ready prepared parcels/presents of familiar and unusual shaped objects in different wrapping paper to develop the discussion further. Encourage the children to guess what is inside each present. Pass it round the group - have more than one parcel being passed round if it is a large group.

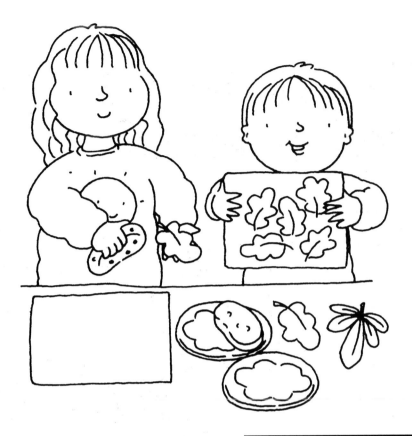

Let them feel it, shake it, explore it but not unwrap it! Such an activity, although simple, develops an awareness of texture and encourages fingers and hands to become more sensitive, making manipulative skills, such as feeding, dressing and pencil control and physical skills, in particular the ability to hold and use tools, much easier. This activity is useful for developing the children's descriptive language, too.

Once the presents have been round the group, place them in a feely box and reinforce the activity by asking the children to take it in turns to choose a present from the box - can they remember what is inside their chosen present?

A theme on presents and in particular the ability to wrap presents is a good way of introducing the children to made materials (boxes and packaging, cardboard, textiles, paper, ribbon, string and wool).

Involve parents by asking the children to bring from home a piece of wrapping paper and if possible the item they would use to secure the wrapping paper. Discuss and display the children's selection of wrapping paper but also show them a variety of other materials which could be used:

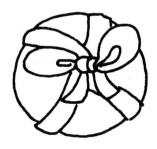

wallpaper, newspaper, computer paper, tissue paper and fabric.

Start wrapping!

For most children, wrapping a present will involve using sticky tape, but encourage them to think of other items which could be used such as glue, staples, string or ribbon and elastic bands.

Once they have the resources they can begin to wrap! Listen to the children's ideas. Whatever solutions they come up with you will need to offer support without telling them what to do as they put their approach into practice - children have imaginations, so let them use them! Through exploration, trial and error they will learn what works and what doesn't. Support the child by explaining or naming unfamiliar materials, extending ideas and keeping up motivation. Make sure there is enough material for each child and replenish the stock when necessary.

What you need:
Paper and card: white, black, coloured paper
Wallpaper (rolls and sample books)
Cardboard and thin card
Tissue paper
Crepe paper
Sticky paper
Kitchen foil
Wrapping paper
Newspaper
Selection of scissors including left-handed ones.
Selection of glue: water paste, PVA glue, glue sticks, flour paste.
Other items: sticky tape, masking tape, stapler and staples, rubber bands, paper clips, string and ribbon and Blu-Tack.

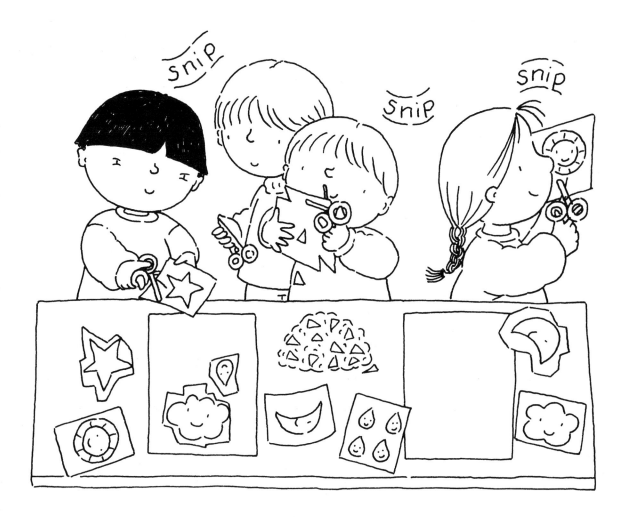

For the child who perhaps lacks the confidence, motivation or ability to work alone then encourage the children to work in small groups with an adult more directly involved.

Provide a range of materials suitable for all abilities and ages, for example glue brushes and glue spatulas - brushes are much easier to use than spatulas. Children may find using larger boxes easier than smaller ones.

Allow the children enough time to complete the activity!

When you first introduce the activity allow the children to explore all the materials you have provided.

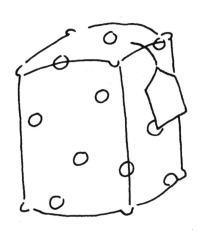

For example, a child may focus on the glue. For adults, glue is used to achieve an end, but for very young children it is an end in itself and encourages them to engage in activities requiring hand-eye coordination. Let them find out about this material that they will use time and time again during their school years. Many children want to know what glue does before they begin to use it for something. Glue can be thick, lumpy, runny, coloured and slimy. There are different types of glue - wallpaper paste, flour paste, paper paste, PVA glue and glue sticks. Let

Other activities

❑ Decorating finished parcels with collage materials. (Creative Development)

❑ To share how they wrapped their presents and what they used. (Language and Literacy)

❑ Printing their own wrapping paper. (Creative Development)

❑ Weighing parcels ready for posting. (Mathematics)

them spread it on their fingers or dribble it down their hands. Provide black paper and give them the opportunity to dribble it onto the paper. What happens when the glue dries? When they are ready, introduce brushes, spatulas and lolly sticks. Slowly through experience and practice they will begin to want to use the glue to stick something together.

Other materials to use in isolation at this stage would be boxes or paper.

Stages 2 and 3 are naturally an extension of stage 1 and the three stages may well overlap. Unlike some of the other activities, this is open-ended so extension activities will depend on and be led by the child. Provide the children with a variety of boxes, card, paper and glue and give them time to explore the materials. They will begin to realise which kind of glue works best in a particular situation, for example light paste works best when using tissue paper but PVA glue is needed for fabric or stiff paper. (You may suggest a simple experiment of using different glues with different materials.)

The children can think of other ways of securing their presents and these materials can be introduced (sticky tape, masking tape, string or ribbon and elastic bands).

You are not looking for a perfectly wrapped present - although this may come in time and with practice.

Scissor skills

To wrap their present the children may have to be able to cut and use scissors appropriately. You may have to help them, perhaps even doing the cutting for them but noting this and planning for scissor skills work in a future session. Encourage and explain the correct use of scissors and help the

children understand how to use them safely as well as how to move around safely when holding or putting scissors away. Similarly, the children may have difficulty in tying string or ribbon. Again, give the children the opportunity to use these items but include in future planning.

As they start to wrap, discuss with the children their choice of wrapping paper. Why did they choose it? Is it easy to use? It may be that some wrapping papers are easier to use and handle than others. Display all their finished presents, whatever they look like!

The older child working at stage 3 may understand the need for careful folding of the ends of the paper. Perhaps ask them to demonstrate this to a younger child. For the older child, provide unusually shaped items to wrap. Why is it much harder to wrap

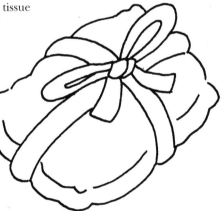

these items? How could they overcome this problem?

Invite someone in from a local department store whose job it is to wrap gifts. The children will be fascinated by how quickly and efficiently it can be done!

Books

A Present for Mum Joan Solomon (Hamish Hamilton).

Gifts and Almonds Joan Solomom (Hamish Hamiton).

Surprises for Presents Hilary Evans (Dinosaur Publications).

Handling construction materials

Young children love familiarity and a theme on Homes and Houses is one all the children, including the youngest, can take part in, as however different their homes may be, they all have one!

Learning objectives

The learning objectives for these activities are endless but could focus on encouraging the children to:

❑ Explore and use items used to build a house.

❑ Play imaginatively to build their own house.

❑ Develop fine motor skills through using a wide range of materials, tools and resources.

All these objectives will easily encourage the children to 'handle tools, objects, construction and malleable materials safely and with increasing control'. (ELG 8)

The learning environment should be well organised and complement your theme and planned activities.

❑ Create a building corner with a variety of bricks of differing shape and size, which the children can use to construct their house.

❑ Create an imaginary building site with sand, water and real and miniature items (bricks, drainpipe, tiles, wheelbarrows, spades and buckets).

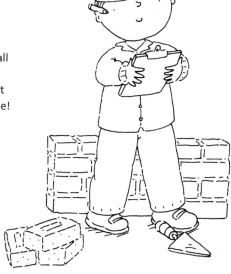

❑ Set up a small play construction site in the sand tray.

Getting started

A good introduction may be to read a story, for example *The House that Jack Built* by Julia Rout or *Tilly's House* by Faith Jaques. This will help the children think about their own homes.

Before introducing this theme to my group I took a photo of each child's house. The photos were used at the introductory session. The children enjoyed finding their house. Having a photo helped them to focus their thoughts and provide correct answers to questions rather than guesses. Staff were able to ask specific questions. For example, 'What colour is your front door?', ' How many windows do you have?' And initial comparisons between the children's homes could begin.

For older children you may still want to use photos, but discussion can be more

detailed - looking at the shape of the windows, doors or roofs or looking at the materials used to build the house.

Another good introduction is to have a feely box containing materials used to build a house (piping, bricks, tiles, sand and wood). In turn children can feel in the box and identify an item. If this is too difficult, young children can remove an item and match it to a similar item on the table.

Older children could make a list beforehand of all the materials they can think of that are needed to build a house. Such an activity encourages physical development by raising awareness of texture and helps fingers and hands to become more sensitive.

Building with sand

The first stage will focus on exploring the materials provided. Children need to go through the stage of tactile exploration before progressing to more formal fine motor skills. The ideal malleable material to use for this theme is sand. The first response to sand is a sensuous one, with children taking pleasure in the tactile experience. However, it also allows children to create and destroy in a safe and acceptable way.

Sand reacts differently when dry, damp or saturated with water and children need the opportunity to explore all three states. Initial free play should focus on encouraging hand exploration, touching, patting,

Small construction

Provide equipment which:

❑ Is versatile and open-ended

❑ Consists of a variety of shapes and sizes which can be combined in an infinite number of ways

❑ Takes account of the physical control of all the children

❑ Has enough pieces for all children

❑ Contains parts such as levers, axles, wheels, and other moving parts

❑ Consists of several construction kits offering the children a choice

holding, pouring and pushing the sand. If damp, the children can mould it as they wish, filling up containers or smoothing it down. These early activities can be extended by providing appropriate equipment to build with - buckets of all sizes, other containers, yoghurt pots, beakers, saucepans and commercially produced items, including plastic brick moulds.

Once they have explored all the items fully, extend their experiences by sensitive adult intervention and questioning. Compare the use of wet/dry sand. Which is the best to build with and why? Can the children build one item on top of another? Can they explain why they cannot? Discussion may move to focus on what builders use to keep bricks together. Why can't they just use sand? What do they have to add to the sand?

Using bricks

The activities at the second stage or later stepping stones can be centred on using bricks. Have a selection of bricks, including real house bricks and play bricks of all shapes and sizes. Encourage the children to really look at the bricks. Can they see the patterns in the house bricks? If it's appropriate, perhaps they can take brick rubbings, which can later be displayed alongside the bricks to provide a matching game.

At first, let the children build with the bricks without adult constraints or suggestions. Construction activities are closely linked with practical maths. When building the children have to estimate the number of bricks required and they are making 3-d shapes and considering size and the necessary pieces needed. Observe the structures the children build. What shapes are chosen? How are they combined? Do the structures show emerging patterns or symmetry? Are the children building vertically, for example towers, or horizontally, for example walls or trains?

Use the children's structures to extend their skills. Do they need to appreciate that bricks are placed in a certain way to add strength? Refer them back to the photographs or look at walls around school if necessary. Can they see that the bricks overlap and interlock? Such discussions can prompt work on tessellation. Why are bricks the shapes they are? What would happen if bricks were cylindrical in shape?

Remember, too, that the size of the bricks will alter the building process as well as the outcome. You may want to extend the children's construction ability and control by giving them smaller construction pieces to use.

Drawing plans

At the third stage children may be ready for the introduction of 2-d plans. They are building 3-d structures, but do they realise they can create a 2-d plan from their structures? Once they have built their models the adult can suggest drawing a plan of the model. At first you can do the drawing, asking the child what features should be included. Once completed the child can be asked if they recognise their model on paper. Does anything have to be altered? Clipboards and pencils can then be left in the building area and the children encouraged to draw plans

or 'pictures' of their favourite models. The two can later be displayed together. This activity not only encourages increased control but also early drawing abilities. Although these final plans may not resemble the model in the adult's eye, the accompanying discussion will reveal the child's appreciation of the shape in relation to each component.

Assessment

Assessment at the first stage may focus on the following:

❑ The children's manipulative skills - can they choose and use tools appropriately? For example, a spade for digging, a sieve for pouring?

❑ Do they use wet and dry sand correctly and can they explain their choice? For example, wet sand for pouring.

❑ Are they beginning to build with the materials provided?

At the second stage, assessment will focus on observing the following:

❑ Can they use large and small construction equipment?

❑ Are they able to build imaginative structures independently or do they need guidance, either to start or extend their work?

❑ Do they use a range of pieces? (differing shapes, sizes and lengths, bolts and screws)

Assessment at the third stage will focus on more complex skills. It may take the form of reversing the activity. Provide the children with 2-d plans of different structures. The children then have to copy and build a 3-d structure from the plan. The plans can increase in difficulty and complexity.

Using a parachute

Using a parachute is very different from other forms of physical play the children may have previously experienced. It is one of the few physical activities (with the exception of team games, which are usually introduced at a later stage) which is dependent on all the children working together as one group. It requires the children to 'take turns and share fairly, understanding that there is a need for agreed values and code of behaviour'.

Perhaps because it is a group activity, it is one area of physical play which is not so much dependent on skill but on the ability to listen, co-operate and interact with their peers. It is an activity which appeals to all ages and abilities.

Parachute play will give the children the opportunity to be interested, excited and motivated to learn. The sheer size, colour and shape of the parachute makes it exciting and it can therefore open up a whole new world to the child.

Learning objectives

Parachute play lends itself to fulfilling many of the Physical Development Early Learning Goals.

It gives children the opportunity to develop ELGs 1, 2, 3, 4 and 8:

❑ Move with confidence, imagination and safety.

❑ Move with control and co-ordination.

❑ Show their awareness of space, of themselves and of others.

❑ Travel around, under and over.

❑ Handle objects with increasing control.

All of these goals are important but, above all, parachute play is an opportunity to work together as part of a group and to have fun!

Organisation

The size of the group will depend on the size of the parachute. Whilst it may be nice to work with the whole group, young children may need a smaller parachute and therefore a smaller group. A smaller parachute is easier to handle and lift off the ground so better for co-operation and interpersonal skills. With young children it is also better to begin with short sessions full of contrasting activities to keep their concentration.

The number of staff or adults available may also dictate the size of the group. Perhaps you could encourage parents or volunteers to join in with the parachute sessions? If you are able to do this, giving the volunteers a simple introduction to the rules or format of the activity before the session may be a good idea. This makes management of the session easier because the lead adult can focus solely on implementing the session and not have to worry about encouraging or controlling the whole group. This allows the session to flow without interruption.

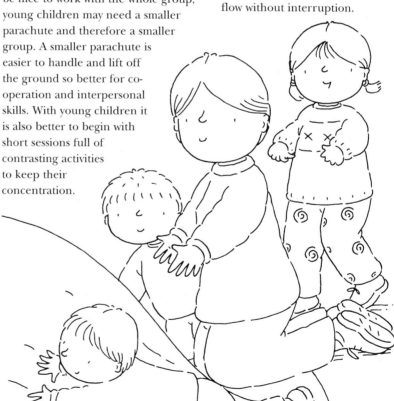

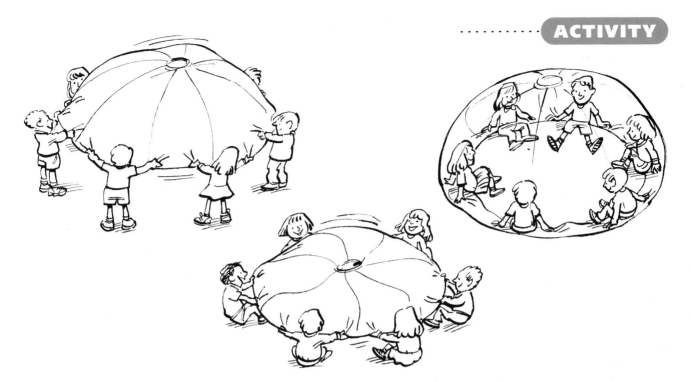

You need the right environment for parachute play. Try to use it in a large space, giving children the opportunity to develop spatial awareness. A confined space means children have to concentrate on not bumping into things rather than enjoying the parachute play. If possible work in an environment where the noise level does not matter! This should be one activity where children are given the freedom to express their emotions.

Parachute play lends itself to use with a mixed ability class. A less confident or less able child can work near an adult in the circle who can encourage and support them.

Looking after your parachute

A parachute is a robust resource if handled correctly. If used correctly it will not tear even under the strain of supporting a child's body weight. Teach the children to respect the parachute:

❑ No pulling, dragging or snatching

❑ No treading on the parachute

❑ Hold it by the handles

❑ Use with an adult

It is difficult to create three clear stages for this activity. Instead I have tried to show progression through extension activities.

Initial sessions at stage 1 will focus on exploring the parachute. Most children will not have worked with a parachute or such a large piece of equipment before. (ELG 7) Encourage them to get the parachute out of its bag - can they lay it flat on the floor?

What is it? Young children may need to be told what it is and it may be an advantage to have pictures or photographs of parachutes in action. Can they guess how large it is? What other objects are as big? Older children could be asked what they could do with the parachute. Let them take the lead and try them out - do their ideas work? If they do, why? And if not, why not? In this way the children will 'interact with each other, negotiate plans and take turns in conversation'. They will also begin to see that parachute work is dependent on teamwork. At a later stage, when the children have some experience of how the parachute moves, it may be appropriate to return to these initial ideas and see if the children can now expand on them to produce more successful ideas.

For the activities the children need to understand the following opposites: up/down; in/out; slow/fast; high/low.

You might decide to take one set of opposites and work on those for several sessions or include a selection of opposites in each session.

The children must realise that the parachute can be manipulated whilst standing up or sitting down. For children who are unable to stand unaided, activities can solely consist of sitting down activities or the child can be supported from behind by an adult.

Standing up activities

Focus at first on the children's attempts at lifting the parachute off the ground. Start by placing the parachute on the floor. The children can stand in a circle around the parachute. When told, the children take hold of the parachute, spacing themselves out. (With young children this may need to be practised and repeated!) Perhaps show them how important it is to be spaced evenly by asking them all to stand very close together on one side of the parachute - they will quickly understand the need for even spacing! Being able to judge space in relation to the space available is an important but early stepping stone. As children develop they should be able to move their body position when requested.

Ask the children to pull the parachute taut and to raise it up as far as they can and then bring it down again. Repeat, trying to get the parachute higher. Once the children have mastered up and down, try the following activities:

❑ Vary the speed of movement, asking them to raise the parachute as fast or as slow as they can. Maybe move it fast as it goes up and slow on the way down.

❑ Start by getting a rhythm of up and down established, then call out the names of two children. They run under the parachute into the centre and back out again, trying to do so before it falls down on them! Some children just love the parachute to fall on them and there is no reason to discourage this but be careful of the less confident child who may be reluctant to be caught underneath.

Alternatively, when their names are called the children have to switch places with one another. At a later stage you can number the children 1-2-3. Then call out one of the numbers and all the children with that number run underneath.

Further progression for those children at stage 3 involves extending the game to the point where more and more children move underneath the parachute. The way in which the children move can also progress. You could call out actions, for example - fly underneath, hop underneath. In

Parachutes can be obtained from most early years catalogues. They come in two different sizes and prices start at around £60. The smaller version is for groups of around 10 children and the larger version for groups of 20 to 30 children. They have strong handles and are made of nylon which allows them to float easily.

this way the children begin to 'travel around and under with increased control and co-ordination'. (ELG 2, 3)

❑ For older children or after several parachute sessions, when the children are competent at moving the parachute up and down, a ball (or several balls) can be placed on top of the parachute. Move the ball(s) backwards and forwards by gently moving the parachute up/down. This requires control and co-ordination because if the parachute is lifted too high the ball(s) will roll off.

For those children who are able to do this encourage them to try and roll the ball around the edge of the taut parachute by moving it in such a way as to achieve a smooth continuous motion.

❑ This time begin the up and down sequence but, once established, when the parachute is at its highest point, the adult shouts 'Let go!' Children love to watch the parachute fall to the ground. If they feel confident, suggest that the children run underneath, allowing the parachute to fall over them. At a later stage the children will come to realise that if they are all able to let go of the parachute at the same time it will stay in the air before coming down.

Sitting down activities

All the standing up activities can be attempted from a sitting position. Using the parachute and sitting down can take two forms.

Everyone sits on the floor with the parachute outstretched and their legs underneath it (that is the children are outside the parachute). The activities can proceed as before. Obviously when sitting down the children will not achieve the height they did when

Assessment

Assessment for this activity will not necessarily be easy unless you are fortunate to have another adult who can sit and observe the group without taking part. You may therefore choose not to assess but just enjoy the activity! For those of you who feel it is important to assess the activity, then assessment can focus on:

❑ The child's ability to understand directional instructions such as up/down or high/low.

❑ The child's control and co-ordination in managing the parachute.

standing up. Activities 2 and 4 in the last section can still be attempted but the children may have to move faster to get underneath when changing places. They may find themselves moving in a different way, perhaps crawling rather than running underneath. Sitting down activities can be less boisterous and can be used at the end of a session or when you want a quieter time. Ask the children to gently move the parachute up and down to make waves.

This time the children sit in a circle under the parachute. They have to hold the parachute from behind and pull it down so they are sitting on it. If this is done immediately after the children have lifted it into the air, pulling it taut and then lowering it to the ground, it will create a large bubble over the children. Once inside the time can be used to relax or to listen to a short story.

A good activity to finish the session with is to ask the children to lie on their tummies in a circle - the adults then move the parachute up and down. Can the children feel the movement of it over their bodies? After a time the parachute can gently be released and allowed to cover the children. Encourage them to be as quiet as possible at this stage.

Make your own parachute

If you don't have a parachute you can always improvise and have fun with a simple sheet or follow the directions here to make your own parachute canopy.

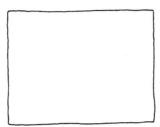

1. Start with an old sheet.

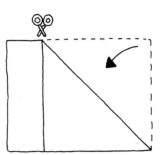

2. Fold as indicated and cut off surplus sheet.

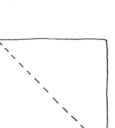

3. Open out to form a square.

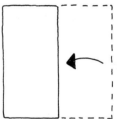

4. Fold once.

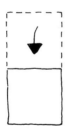

5. Fold again to form a small square.

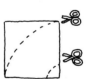

6. Draw lines as indicated.

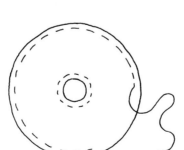

7. Open out to form the canopy. Hem to strengthen.

8. Add handles if required.

Fun activities for two

❑ Give a favourite teddy a ride by sitting it in the middle of the sheet, holding the sides and lifting them up and down to make the teddy bounce.

❑ Roll a soft ball around on the sheet and try to get it through the hole in the middle.

Activities for two or three children

❑ Let two children hold up the sheet while the third crawls underneath.

❑ Ask a child to sit in the middle of the sheet and get the other two to flap the sides.

❑ Have one child lying under the sheet while the others roll a ball around on the sheet above. See if the child can kick or punch the ball off the sheet from underneath.

Idea supplied by Jean Evans, early years inspector and consultant
(First published in *Practical Pre-School* Issue 18, November 1999.)

Physical
Development

Developing ball skills

Give a child a ball and they will immediately do something with it. They may throw it, bounce it, kick it or just hang on to it! It can be whatever they want it to be - a magic ball, a giant lollipop or a flying saucer.

Manipulative skills, which involve gross motor movements, can be classed as ball skills - throwing, catching and kicking. Ball skills not only involve the use of small equipment (ELG 7) but they also develop a child's ability to control and co-ordinate body actions (ELG 2). They develop an awareness of the space they are working in as they judge speed and distance when throwing or kicking the ball (ELG 4).

Learning objectives

The learning objectives focus on these three Early Learning Goals (2, 4, 7):

❑ To move with control and co-ordination.

❑ To show an awareness of space, of themselves and of others.

❑ To use a range of small and large equipment.

Getting started

The starting point for these activities may be simply to give the children each a ball. Allow them the freedom to do what they want with it. (Obviously this is easier and safer if you are outside in a large space!) Give them the time and opportunity to use the ball whilst you stand back and observe what they can do. This can inform future planning. When their interest begins to wane, ask them to try some different activities. Can they bounce the ball? Can they kick the ball? Can they throw the ball? Can they hold onto the ball and run?

Introduce the children to a variety of balls - soft and hard, large and small. In this way they will begin to see that the type of ball influences what can be done with it.

You are aiming to help children adopt skills and abilities that will enable them to join in a range of activities. Ball skills follow a developmental pattern, so I have divided the activities into three sections - throwing, catching and kicking. Each section briefly shows the progression within each skill and gives some ideas for promoting the skill.

Throwing

Children are able to throw from an early age! However, it is several years before they develop enough co-ordination to have control over the direction in which the object is thrown. (ELG 2)

Children need practice in throwing or pushing a range of objects (balls, bean bags, quoits and hoops). To begin with, this will also include practising throwing objects without falling over! Children then progress to being able to throw at body level, then overhand and underhand. Once they have mastered this, they can throw to a

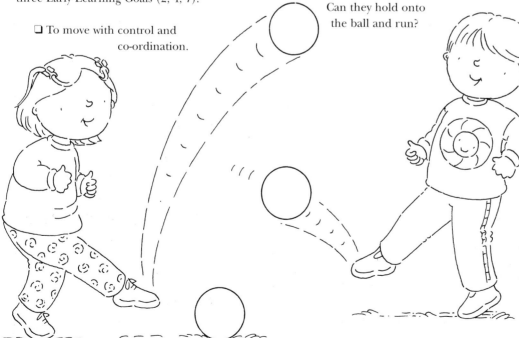

partner, throw an object into a bucket, hoop or net (ELG 7). Encourage them to try and throw and knock down a target, for example a cone or wicket. How far can each child throw? Who can throw the furthest?

Games can be introduced but not too soon. Wait until the children are able to co-operate with each other in physical play and understand the need for turn taking and negotiating.

Catching

The ability to catch a ball often comes later than being able to throw a ball. Only children who are working at a later stepping stone will have the control and manipulation to use a ball appropriately. At first, children tend to use their outstretched arms and body to catch the ball. With poor co-ordination and timing they often miss the ball and success is usually due to the thrower rather than the catcher! With practice they will be able to catch the ball with their hands and body before progressing to be able to catch using their hands only. Children should be given a range of objects to use to practise this skill. Objects such as balloons, bean bags and quoits may be easier.

When the children are ready, introduce a range of balls which differ in size and in type. The speed at which a ball is thrown also makes a difference. At first the thrower should throw quite slowly but, as the child's skill develops, then the speed of the thrown ball can increase.

Once the children are consistently catching balls, they can work in pairs. Give each pair several balls. One child begins and throws the balls to the other child. Encourage them to count and keep score of the number of balls the catcher is able to catch. Once all the balls have been thrown the children can swap roles. Once they are proficient, ask the thrower to throw so

that the catcher has to reach down low or reach up to catch the ball.

Games to develop catching and throwing skills

Have the children standing in a circle. Encourage them to throw the ball gently from one child to another as it's passed round the circle. Make it more difficult. This time the child with the ball calls out the name of another child and throws the ball to them across the circle. Increasing the distance like this helps to improve hand-eye co-ordination and hand control.

The children remain in a circle. One child stands in the middle. As the children throw the ball to each other across the circle, the child in the middle has to try and catch it or pick it up when it is dropped. If he is successful, he changes places with the last child to handle the ball.

Again, the children stand in a circle with one child in the centre. This time the child in the middle has control of the ball. He throws it to a child in the outer circle who runs with the ball round the circle, back to his place and once there throws it back to the child in the middle who then throws it to the next child, and so on.

The children are in two teams standing in lines the length of the hall or room. At one end of the line the first child in each team is given a ball. When the adult says 'Go!', each team has to throw and catch the ball down the line. Which team can get their ball to the other end of the room first?

Kicking

Kicking is a difficult skill, particularly if the ball is moving. It involves co-ordinating the speed and direction of the ball as well as co-ordinating the body to kick the ball. For many children within the Foundation Stage you will be working on stationary

kicking - you will not be expecting them to move and kick simultaneously. This skill can be encouraged in a number of ways. How far can each child kick? Can they kick and hit a target? Can they kick it to another child? (ELG 2, 4)

When the children are ready, have two teams of children, one team at each end of the room. Encourage them to kick the ball between teams. Begin with a short distance between each team and gradually make it longer and longer.

Assessment

As this is a skill-based activity, the assessment is presented as a check-list. You may choose to assess in a different way.

Ball skills

❑ Rolls a ball

❑ Throws or kicks a ball without falling

❑ Throws a ball at body level

❑ Throws a ball overhand

❑ Throws a ball underhand

❑ Catches a ball - arms and body

❑ Catches a ball - hands and body

❑ Catches a ball - hands only

❑ Able to kick or throw to another person

❑ Able to participate in organised games - football, rounders and cricket

---

Books

Games In and Out Roundabout Gillian Ellis (Printforce Publication).

Let's Play these Games Francis Lane (Printforce Publication).

Healthy eating:
The Very Hungry Caterpillar

The story of 'The Very Hungry Caterpillar' will be familiar to many children and adults working within the Foundation Stage. It is a good story, with lots of repetition and a clear sequence of events. It lends itself to mathematical work linked to the days of the week and descriptive language of shape and size. The story can also be used to encourage the children to identify features of living things and look closely at the change from caterpillar to butterfly. However, it is also a useful story for promoting physical development, encouraging the children to recognise the importance of keeping healthy and the things which contribute to this. The activities below focus on healthy eating as one way of keeping healthy.

Learning objectives

The main learning objective is to fulfil the ELG for health and bodily awareness (ELG 5):

❏ To recognise the importance of keeping healthy and those things which contribute to this.

Throughout the activities the children will also be expected:

❏ To listen to and retell the story in their own words.

Getting started

The starting point for the activities is the story itself. Even with very young children it will probably be appropriate to read the story to the whole group. The activities that follow involve discussion, cookery and craft. These activities may be more manageable and the children able to take a more active part if they are carried out in smaller groups with an adult working with each group. Not all settings will be able to accommodate this. If not, then have one small group working with an adult involved in supporting activities, while the rest of the group are independently involved in a range of related activities (see 'Other activities') which do not require continual adult support.

Within all stepping stones, read the story first. Read it more than once, encouraging the children to listen the first time it is read, but then inviting them to help you retell the story with you. At stage 1, the children will probably still need you and the book to help them, but they should be beginning to answer questions about where, why and how.

Prepare pictures of the food the caterpillar eats. (Laminate them to make them more durable.) Use these pictures for a simple sorting activity. At stages 2 and 3 you may expect the children to be beginning to retell stories in the correct sequence and show an understanding of the elements of the story. They should be able to identify the main character (the caterpillar) and the sequence of events

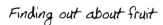

(the days of the week) and what he eats on each day. One way of encouraging and promoting this is to ask the children to use the food pictures from stage 1. On separate, individual cards have the days of the week. Can the children place the food pictures under the appropriate day? (Particularly in the early part of the week, when the caterpillar is eating lots of fruit, this activity would also fulfil many of the mathematical ELGs.)

Finding out about fruit

Discussion can follow the story and should be linked to healthy eating. At the early stages, begin by discussing what fruit the caterpillar ate and how many of each fruit? Ask the children what fruit they eat. Which is their favourite? Explain that fruit is good for us. Do they know why? List their answers for future reference.

Encourage the children to appreciate the variety of skin coverings, textures, colour and sizes of the fruit by introducing a feely box. Place the fruit in the box. Invite the children to be blindfolded and ask them to remove one piece of fruit. Encourage them to feel and touch the fruit before attempting to name it. (This requires good manipulative skill as they carefully handle the fruit.) Can they describe its texture and its shape? This is a good activity not only for

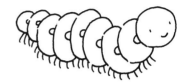

encouraging a sense of touch but also descriptive language. Once the children have all had a go, turn the activity round and make it more difficult. Ask the children to find a smooth fruit or a furry fruit. Perhaps move on to a similar activity but this time when the children are blindfolded invite them to taste the fruit. Can they tell what they are eating?

Encourage the children to appreciate the range of fruit by asking them to bring in one piece of fruit from home. Display (or taste) each fruit. (Some supermarkets go into settings to give talks about exotic fruit and take samples with them.) Remember continually to place the discussion in the context of keeping healthy and remind the children that staying healthy consists of healthy eating, staying active and resting well.

Further activities could include making special fruit dishes, for example, fruit salad and fruit fool. You could do some fruit printing and display the paintings around photos and pictures of the fruit. Both these activities continue to raise an awareness of healthy eating but also encourage increased control in handling tools (ELG 8) and promoting hand-eye co-ordination.

Stages 2 and 3

At stages 2 and 3 the discussion following the story should be more in-depth. As at stage 1, look at the food the caterpillar eats. Using pictures of all the foods, ask the children to divide the foods into two groups - 'good' food and 'bad' food. Which group do they put each food in and can they explain why? Why is fruit good for us but cake and salami not so good? If they are able, subdivide the groups in a different way, into four groups: bread and cereal; milk and dairy; fruit and vegetables; and meat, fish, eggs and nuts. Have a selection of other foods and encourage the children to paste

the pictures under the appropriate heading. (Begin to emphasise the importance of a balanced diet for healthy living and not over-indulging - like the caterpillar.) What made the caterpillar ill? What foods should they eat in moderation and why? The story follows the caterpillar's food intake over one week. Encourage the children to keep a food diary for a week. (They can draw what they eat - or cut out pictures - instead of writing.) Then spend time looking at the diaries. What are the similarities and differences? Are they able to identify the foods that aren't so good for them? What could they eat instead of these things? Staff, too, should keep a diary. Ask the children to tell you what food you are eating that isn't healthy. Such activities should help children, particularly those working within the later stepping stones, to understand the importance of a good eating pattern.

At these stages the children could make observational drawings of real fruit (ELG 8) or perhaps make a feely caterpillar from old tights or socks.

Fruit week

If the children regularly bring snacks to school, then for one week encourage them to bring only fruit. Keep a tally of the number of different fruits they bring in. At the beginning of the week, ask them to guess how many different fruits will be brought in.

Books

Each Peach, Pear, Plum Janet and Allan Ahlberg (Viking Kestrel).

The Shopping Basket John Burningham (Cape).

Fruit Graham Houghton (*Focus on* series, Wayland).

Fruit Salad: A First Look at Fruit Julia Eccleshare (Hamish Hamilton).

Other activities

These are activities that the children could be involved in alongside the teacher directed ones outlined above.

Stage 1

❑ Fruit lotto or fruit inset puzzles. (Mathematical/Physical Development)

❑ Making caterpillars using cotton reels on lacing threads. (Physical Development)

Stage 2/3

❑ Creating butterfly prints. (Mathematical Development/ Creative Development)

❑ Modelling fruit using salt dough. (Physical Development/ Creative Development)

At all stages set up a cafe or fruit and vegetable shop in the imaginative play area. (Communication, Language and Literacy/Creative Development)

Assessment

I have decided not to assess this theme, mainly because the idea of healthy eating is a personal thing, something the children have to do for themselves. It is our role to encourage and promote it but ultimately it has to be a child's decision to follow a healthy lifestyle.

How our bodies work

In all the movement activities you offer the children, you should be helping the children feel good about themselves and their bodies. The Scottish curriculum framework document emphasises that a child's growing confidence and enjoyment of physical play influences their physical development. You need to help them with this by creating a positive attitude towards physical activities and offering activities which ensure success as well as progression. Respecting our bodies is part of feeling good about ourselves. Children need to be encouraged to look after themselves by eating well, staying active, having a good sleep and keeping clean.

Learning objectives

Children are able to:
❑ Recognise the changes that happen to their bodies when they are active. (ELG 6)

Getting started

A good starting point is a discussion centred on 'Our bodies'. Obviously the level of discussion will depend on the age of the children, their abilities and their backgrounds. Some may be young but come from families where exercise and a balanced diet forms a regular part of family life. An older child may have more limited understanding of the need to stay healthy and how their body works because they rarely exercise outside of school.

Before children can recognise the changes that take place in their bodies as a result of physical activity, they need to have some understanding of their

bodies at rest as well as understanding a little of how the body works and the parts it is made up of.

At all stages discussion can begin by asking the children what they need in order to move.

Young children will probably focus on large body parts such as arms, legs or feet. Even at this stage, though, encourage them to think of the internal body parts they may be using, such as blood, heart, lungs and muscles. Emphasise the need for all the parts, both inside and out, to work together to keep their bodies moving.

For children at stage 1, ask one of them to lie on the floor. Draw round them to produce a body outline. Repeat this with another child. Then using the two body shapes, together with the children begin to create an 'inside man' and an 'outside woman'. On each outline draw and write the body parts the children are talking about.

Once the children are able to name some body parts, particularly the internal ones, they need to begin to understand how each part works and what it does. You will know the children you are working with and so will be able to gauge just how detailed the explanations should be. I have given explanations for two stages and these should be used as a guide only.

Stage 1

For younger children you may focus on:

Muscles: Emphasise that muscles help us move - to run, walk, sit or lie down.

We need them and use them for big and little actions, for example kicking a ball or picking up a pencil. Can the children show you where their muscles are? What muscles would they use for running or drawing?

Heart: Do they know where their heart is? For young children it may be enough for them to understand that the heart beats all the time but when they are running or doing other physical activities it starts to beat faster.

Stage 2

For older or more able children discussion may be more detailed and include:

Heart: Explain that the heart works all the time. Just as an engine needs petrol or fuel to keep going, our bodies need fuel too. The heart pumps blood around our bodies, taking oxygen, which is the fuel, to the cells of the body to give us energy to do things. Each pump of the heart is called the heart beat. Ask the children to press their fingers down inside their wrists. Can they feel their wrist throbbing? Do they know what the throbbing is called? Do they know what happens to their heart rate when they run around and exercise? Do they know why?

Lungs: Explain to the children that without their lungs they would be unable to blow up a balloon, shout or breathe. Lungs act like two giant sponges, soaking up oxygen from the air. Oxygen is the useful part of the air we breath. We take in air through our nose and mouth; it goes down our throat into our lungs where it fills up the air sacs. The lungs then take the oxygen into the blood and the blood is pumped round the body by the heart to our cells, which need the oxygen in order to work. Can the children tell you what happens to their pulse or breathing rate after exercise? Why does this happen?

For the children to appreciate how their bodies work, they need to put into practice the things they have been discussing. At the beginning of the activity have the children together in a large group. At stage 1, give them time to be still. Remind them of the things you have discussed. What parts of their bodies are they about to use? Encourage them to focus on how they are feeling when at rest, for example, their breathing is steady, they feel quiet, relaxed, and calm.

For children at stages 2 and 3, asking them to take their pulse and breathing rates can reinforce the discussion. Once they have exercised, both rates can be taken again. What are the differences? What has caused the differences and why? Keep a record of all the children's rates. Over a term or year do they change? If they do, why might that be?

The exercises can be of your choosing and linked to the needs of the children in your group. It may be appropriate to have a mixture of activities, for example hopping, skipping and jumping (see pages 9-10 for ideas on the progression in these areas) and team activities focusing on running. The aim of the activities is to increase cardiovascular rates, so make sure the activities involve speed and changing direction frequently! Using music is a good way of doing this. Either use the music and give children the opportunity to move and dance freely or use it to support action songs such as 'The Grand Old Duke of York' or 'The Hokey Cokey' - both involve energetic movements. Music is also useful at the end of a session as part of a cool-down or relaxation activity.

The discussion which follows the activity is as important as the physical exercise itself.

Children at stage 1 should begin to recognise that after exercise they are beginning to feel tired but good, hot and sticky, their hearts are beating faster and they now want to rest. They may feel the need to have a drink or something to eat.

Children at stages 2 and 3 who take their pulse and breathing rates after exercise will begin to recognise the physiological changes that take place within their bodies during exercise. The role of the adult at both stages is to extend and encourage the children's ideas and answers. To reinforce the importance of keeping healthy and to correct any misconceptions, children also need to understand that their bodies work more efficiently if they look after themselves. Discuss healthy eating and the importance of diet (see pages 42-43 for further ideas on this theme) as well as the importance of rest and sleep.

Assessment

If we are aiming to promote a healthy lifestyle and encourage children to be involved in taking more exercise then they have to be in control. For this reason, I would suggest that the assessment for this activity should be child-led.

Give the children their own charts, rather like star charts (see below). Encourage the children to complete the chart either by sticking on a smiley face - one face for each time they have done some exercise (perhaps more appropriate for younger children) - or by writing in the activity or exercise. The charts could be shared and discussed within the group or you may feel it is more appropriate for the children to keep the charts to themselves.

My exercise chart

Exercise	Monday	Tuesday	Wednesday	Thursday	Friday	Saturday	Sunday
	☺						

Finding your pulse

Show children how they can feel their pulse in the hollow alongside the outer bone of their wrist.

They need to press firmly but gently with two fingers.

Count the number of beats they feel in one minute.
(You'll need to time them.)

What do they think will change this rate?

Counting your breathing rate

Ask children to try to behave as naturally as possible.

Explain that when they count their breathing rate, they should count each time they breathe in, ignoring the times they breathe out.

See if they can count the number of times they breathe in one minute. Record this result.

Keeping healthy

One of the Physical Development Early Learning Goals is aimed at promoting health and bodily awareness. Children need to recognise the importance of keeping healthy and those things which contribute to this.

A theme on 'Keeping healthy', though, must be set in context. A setting or school which promotes good health not only makes children aware of the need to look after themselves but also provides a healthy environment in which children can work or play. For example, it is no good teaching the children that too much sugar is harmful for teeth or weight if sweets are regularly used as rewards for good work or allowed in lunch boxes. You and your staff need to ask some searching questions, for example, is the food you provide at snack time healthy? Do you encourage the children to take regular exercise both in and outside of school? Are meals nutritional and well balanced with a good choice? Are parents encouraged to take part in the curriculum?

Good health means looking after yourself - eating well, staying active, keeping clean and having a good night's sleep. It also means learning to feel good about yourself, valuing others and feeling responsible for your environment.

Learning objective

The aim of these activities is for the children to recognise both the importance of keeping healthy and those things which contribute to it - exercise, healthy eating, sleep. (ELG 5, 6)

Starting point

A good starting point for this theme would be for the children to build up a picture of themselves that they can begin to feel proud of.

Ask each child to find out how much they weigh, how tall they are and what size clothes and shoes they take. For children at stage 1 this can be done as a group and the information recorded through bar or pie charts. You might draw round each child; they could then paint or collage their outlines and display them in correct order of size.

Children at stage 2 could be encouraged to complete the work at home and then bring it in to show everyone. The information could be used to produce their own concertina 'All about me' books.

Children at stage 3 can discuss what factors contribute to height and weight. They might also begin to look at themselves in relation to others. Give them a blank piece of paper and suggest they draw themselves in the centre. Then they can add round the picture, names or pictures of significant people in their lives, helping them to recognise that who we are and what we do is influenced by and influences those around us.

All the children can talk about skin, hair and eye colour. Encourage them to see that we are all different yet have many similarities.

Ask the children to think about the things they are good at. Many children find this difficult so, particularly for older children, let them discuss it in their groups. Often other people can see our good points better than we can! Celebrate their achievements.

Much of this work will be group based with the children working together, giving them the confidence to share ideas and feelings and helping to develop the skills of co-operation and appreciating the needs of others.

Regular exercise

(See also pages 44-45, 'How our bodies work'.) Exercise benefits almost everyone. It improves mood, appetite, quality of sleep and general health. It is, therefore, important to encourage children to use their bodies to the full. They need to be given the chance to move about freely and enjoy a range of physical activities. Are there activities that they can do during breaktimes as well as during planned physical activity sessions?

At all stages you could give the children running, jumping or throwing challenges, designed to encourage use of the whole body, increasing the strength in their arms and legs and helping them to develop control and co-ordination. (ELG 2) Ask the children to see who can run or jump the furthest or fastest. Increase the distance you expect them to run as they get older (emphasising personal success rather than competitiveness).

Try seeing how long they can jump or run for without stopping. Do this at regular intervals throughout the year to build up stamina and encourage the children to see the improvement. Does stamina depend on age?

Healthy eating

(See also pages 42-43, 'Health eating: The Very Hungry Caterpillar'.)

Healthy eating does not mean dieting and it is important to stress this to the children. Instead, you should be helping the children to eat a balanced, healthy diet. This can also be linked with dental hygiene by raising awareness of the link between diet and dental health. You can focus on three aspects:

❑ Reducing sugar intake (which also includes brushing teeth regularly);

❑ Eating a variety of foods;

❑ Increasing intake of fruit and vegetables.

Many children may be eating a relatively healthy diet but fall down on the snacks they have. Start by looking at snacks. Do the children know what we mean by a snack? Children at all stages can begin by compiling a list of the snacks they eat (including drinks). Children at stage 1 can perhaps do this as a group activity with the adult recording their answers. Children at stages 2 and 3 can do the same or perhaps draw up their own lists, which can then be compared with their peers. Discussion can follow. What foods are healthy snacks and good for our teeth? Which are not? Children who are working within the later stepping stones should be able to show some understanding of good practices with regard to eating and good health.

Children enjoy tasting different foods so have a healthy snack session. Foods to include are: crispbreads/crackers and cheese, bread sticks, milkshakes, fruit and vegetable sticks, healthy sandwiches with fillings such as carrot and cheese or tomato and ham, puffed crisps, dried apricots and sultanas,

plain biscuits and dips. Encourage the younger children to name the foods that they are about to try. Older children can be encouraged to explain why the snacks are classed as healthy and why they are better than fizzy drinks, chocolate and sugary biscuits. After tasting, the children can say which snack they liked best and why. Will they try it again at home?

Another idea is to visit a greengrocer's shop. What types of fruit and vegetables are for sale? Pick out those that the children don't know. (Stage 1) Back in your setting, the children can sort a selection into two groups - fruit and vegetables, or perhaps sort by colour or shape. Can they handle the fruit carefully using fine hand control to pick up, touch and describe some of the fruit?

Children at stages 2 and 3 can list as many fruits and vegetables as they can think of. To challenge them further, ask them to think of an apple. How many ways can you eat an apple? (raw, in apple pie, crumble, baked, stewed, chutney, jelly, and so on) Perhaps you could cook some apples together in several ways. Cutting, chopping and mixing the fruit will all involve fine hand control and develop their ability to handle tools appropriately. (ELG 8)

Bring the discussion back to the child's own eating habits. Look at their lunches, either school lunch or a packed lunch. Has anyone brought fruit to school? Make a list of the types of fruit. Explain you will do the same next week. Have more children now brought fruit to school? (Be careful not to be critical or judgmental about the food children have at home.)

Good sleep

We all have different sleeping habits. Some people seem to need more sleep than others. However, children need to recognise how important sleep is. Begin by asking them if they know why

Assessment

As for the theme on 'Healthy eating', assessment is in many ways inappropriate. Instead you need continually to promote a healthy lifestyle in everything that you do. Return to this theme periodically to remind the children of the importance of good health.

it is important. What happens if we don't get enough sleep? Try to involve the parents in this theme. Ask the parents of children at stage 1 to keep a sleep diary for their child for one week, noting down both the bedtime and the time their child got up. Children at later stages can keep their own diaries. Discuss the diaries. Create a bar chart showing bedtimes. Who goes to bed the earliest/latest? What is the most popular bedtime? (This may indicate the time that most parents feel is appropriate.)

Children at stages 2 and 3 can extend the activity. Can they work out how many hours sleep each child has? You can then compare who has the longest/shortest sleep. Is the result affected by the time the child goes to bed? For what reasons are they allowed to stay up later? Hopefully keeping these diaries will help children begin to appreciate why they need to go to bed at a reasonable time.

Other activities

❑ Healthy eating: Create a healthy lunch box with real food or using pictures. (Physical Development)

❑ Good sleep: Make books showing bedtime routines. (Communication, Language and Literacy)

Book

Planning for Learning through ... All About Me Penny Coltman and Rachel Linfield (Step Forward Publishing).

Physical Development

Seasons

Sorting seeds

Seeds are a natural material and can be used for a variety of activities linked to the theme of spring and new growth. They are a rich resource for developing many of the Early Learning Goals. Through these activities the children will be encouraged to observe and examine the world around them and develop within them a growing awareness of change which is so apparent through the seasons. Encourage the children to look at the similarities and differences within the seasons and in particular the seeds, encouraging them to discover and experiment. Give children opportunities to listen and talk about their experiences.

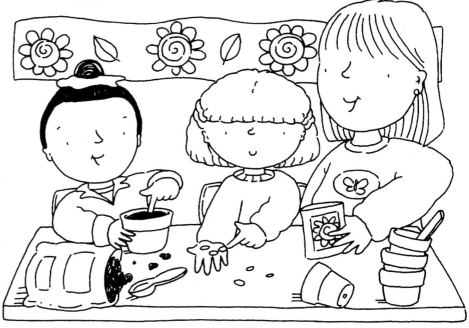

Learning objectives

The learning objectives for these activities are for children:

❏ to examine the world around them and develop a growing awareness of change.

❏ to begin to understand the need for water, light and food in order to sustain growth.

❏ to be able to identify what a seed is, sort a variety of seeds into sets, developing their skills of identification and classification.

As they fulfil these learning objectives, the children will have the opportunity to work with seeds of all shapes and sizes, which will include the use of a range of tools. Handling the seeds and the tools will require the children to have refined hand-eye co-ordination and will help develop increasing control of fine movements of the fingers and hands. (ELG 8)

Getting started

You'll need to collect seeds and seed packets (some garden centres will let you have out-of-date packets). Ask parents to send in one seed packet chosen by their child. Also have a variety of fruits or plants with an abundance of seeds; particularly good examples are oranges, tomatoes, apples, cucumbers, sunflower heads, pomegranates and broad beans.

If it's spring, before you do any sorting, go on a nature walk. Look out for new growth and buds in both the plant and animal world.

Using your collection of seeds and plants, start by asking the children what a seed is. Record their answers on pieces of paper which can later be used for display. Encourage them to give their answers and explanations freely. At stage 1, this may simply be 'It

grows'. At stages 2 and 3 you will be expecting them to understand the concept of growth and change and may well link their answers to things observed on their walk.

Another way of showing change and growth is to read the story of 'The Enormous Turnip'. Have any planted seeds at home? Do they understand what was needed to help the seeds grow? What happens if they are not watered or have too much sun? At stage 1 it may be enough to read the story and follow it up with discussion. For children at stage 2 you may expect them to retell the story, asking them to focus on why the turnip seed grew and grew. What was needed? You could give children at stage 3 pictures showing the stages in growth and see if they can sequence the pictures correctly.

Give all the children the opportunity to explore freely and observe the seeds.

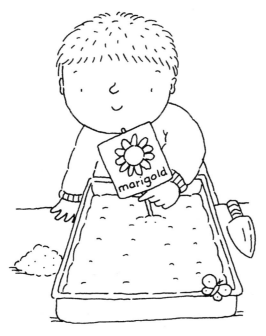

Have the seeds on polystyrene trays or in petri dishes. Talk about the colour, shape and size of the seeds, encouraging the children to note any major similarities and differences between them. Extend the activity by having a selection of cards. Stick one type of seed onto each card and give the children a card each. Can they match the seeds on their cards to seeds in the tray?

Children at stage 3 can be asked to sort and classify the seeds as well. Begin with big seeds and little seeds - which is the biggest in the collection? Such an activity will require sensitive handling and gentle manipulative movements. Ask them to sort the seeds by colour. This should produce some interesting language as the children discuss (and argue!) which seed belongs where!

Handling tools

Give all the children the opportunity to use magnifying glasses and lenses to study the seeds more closely. Show them how to use them appropriately. For children at stage 1, this may be their first introduction to these pieces of equipment. Give them time to use them thoroughly. Children who are more familiar with using them can be asked to choose one or two seeds and, using the equipment, make more detailed observations. These can be recorded in pictorial form. Can they identify which seed packet their chosen seed came from? Remind them that their seeds will grow into the plant or flower on the packet. Can they find out which month the seed will flower? What season is it in? Help the children to draw the plant or flower alongside their seed drawing. Encourage them to label the month the seed should be planted and also the month it will flower. How long do they have to wait?

In a later session the children can be given the opportunity to plant their own seeds. For young children use seeds which grow quickly, such as cress or beans. Watch the changes and record the findings. Older children can plant seeds such as lettuce, onions or tomatoes. These are slower to grow but satisfying to pick to eat later in the year. Alternatively, plant flower seeds in small trays indoors which can be replanted outside when big enough and the weather is warmer.

Looking at flowers

Encourage the children to look at flowers (perhaps even those they have sown in the spring). Can they examine them (handling them carefully) and list all the things that can be said about one particular bloom - its colour, size, shape and texture? Set aside an area for a flower display along with relevant books, magnifying glasses and lenses. Keep the display going throughout the summer, encouraging the children to bring flowers in from home. Can they paint a picture of their flower?

Baking bread

In autumn, you could focus on the Christian festival of Harvest. Explain that harvest is the time to give thanks to God for the safe production of this year's crops. Today this festival is often an opportunity to thank God for all the food we have. One way of celebrating harvest is for the children to eat

something they have grown. Sow cress again and make your own cress sandwiches. You could even make your own bread - kneading dough is a very physical activity and good for strengthening hand muscles.

Books

In the Garden Macdonald *Zero* (Macdonald).

Seeds and Weeds Macdonald *Starters* (Macdonald).

Physical Development

Water

Noah's ark

Young children are fascinated by water. Despite its familiarity, water is a rich resource which children enjoy exploring, investigating and discovering. Through playing in the bath, washing the dolls' clothes, watering the garden or playing in the water tray, the children begin to learn how water behaves, what it can be used for and what we can do with it.

At the earlier stepping stones, as they fill and empty containers, they will be developing the skills of gripping and grasping as well as hand-eye coordination as they pour the water from one container to another.

Their language also develops as they use appropriate vocabulary to describe what is happening.

The ideas for activities centred on the water tray are endless, so instead I have tried to come up with some creative movement activities which link the Water theme to the story of Noah's ark. The ideas could be a series of short sessions which are then brought together or they can be part of a one-off movement session.

There are no stages for this activity. Adapt the ideas to suit your own children.

Learning objectives

The Scottish curriculum framework document suggests that as children respond to their moods, feelings or to music and imaginative ideas they become aware that they can use their bodies to express ideas and feelings by moving in different ways. The activities will also fulfil many of the English goals for Creative Development. This is the focus of these activities. In addition the learning objectives will also be for the children to:

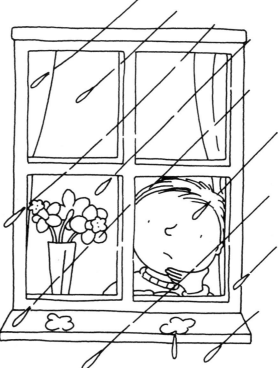

❑ Move with confidence, imagination and in safety. (ELG 1)

❑ Move with control and co-ordination. (ELG 2)

❑ Respond to the story to produce a movement sequence.

Getting started

The starting point for the movement session is the story. Read the story of Noah's ark and then discuss it with the children. Why did God send a flood? Do they know what a flood is? Why do flood disasters happen? Can they be prevented? Why did God save Noah and his family? Talk about the animals in the ark.

You may need to read the story several times for the children to know it well enough to be able to enact it for themselves.

Give your children the freedom to try out their own ideas, as well as mine. The ones below should be seen as suggestions only.

The children sit together in a circle in the hall or large outdoor space.

Pitter, patter, raindrops

The first activity is based on the rain and the flood. Encourage the children to think of the rain and how it poured and poured until there was so much rain that the water covered all the earth.

Ask the children how they could show the rain falling through movement. What body parts could they use? They could begin by using one finger to gently and slowly tap on the floor as the first raindrops appear. One finger could become several fingers as they now drum on the floor to signify the raindrops becoming a shower. As the shower turns to heavy rain, they need to drum harder using either hands or even their feet. Perhaps they could clap their hands several times for thunder, before going back to heavy rain and then back through the rest of the sequence they have just created to

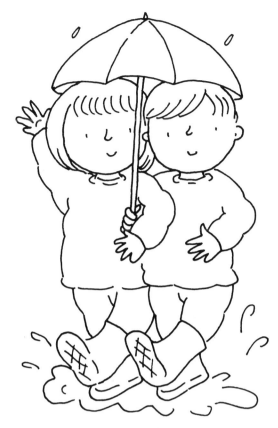

the point where, finally, the rain stops. This idea involves the children working in isolation but they may be able to create a way of working as a whole group to imitate the rain falling.

Later they may want to introduce percussion instruments or ribbons to support their movements in creating the rain effect. By doing so they will be developing their skill at handling tools and objects with increased control. (ELG 8)

The animals went in two by two

The second activity can be linked to the animals that enter the ark. The children could work in pairs for this. They can choose the animal they are going to be. As a pair they will need to know how their particular animal moves. Is the animal slow or fast? Heavy or light? What body parts can they use so that their animal is recognisable? Emphasise the need for movement which shows strength, exaggeration and repetition. Encourage them to use their voices to make appropriate animal sounds as they move. Together they will need to

decide how to move rhythmically. Can they move together without falling over?

Building the ark

The third activity centres on building the ark. This time the children can work as a whole group. This will require them working together, taking turns and sharing, understanding the need for agreed values and for every child's ideas to be treated with respect.

Begin by discussing with the children how they will go about building the ark. What will they be using? How are they going to show the height, length and width of the ark through movement? Record their ideas on large pieces of paper which can then be used as an aide-memoir when creating the sequence.

If you decide to combine all three activities to create a finished piece of dance and movement then the children need to plan for this, taking decisions on who will do what, whether there is to be music, instruments or costumes to support the dance. Who will be the audience? And where will it take place?

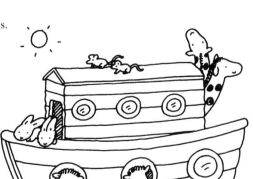

Assessment

Although assessment can be centred around the learning objectives, such an activity interrelates and supports so many other curricular areas, particularly skills relating to Personal, Social and Emotional Development, that it may be more appropriate to video the finished dance and keep it as a record of achievement. If you don't have access to a video camera, take photographs.

Other activities

❑ Water play activities: floating and sinking. (Knowledge and Understanding of the World)

❑ The weather, in particular, measuring rainfall. (Knowledge and Understanding of the World)

❑ Counting the animals and putting into pairs. (Mathematical Development)

❑ Discussing what they would take with them if they were going in the ark. (Communication, Language and Literacy)

Songs, music and stories

'The Animals Went in Two by Two' in *Appuskidu* (A & C Black).

'Who Built The Ark?' in *Someone's Singing Lord* (A & C Black).

Noah and His Ark Retold by Catherine Storr (Franklin Watts).

Come Away From The Water, Shirley John Burningham (Red Fox).

Ribbon games and traffic lights

These activities are designed to reinforce a child's knowledge and ability to name colours through physical activities. The activities progress from easy through to more difficult. The level of difficulty relates to the physical skills expected at each stage and not to the children's ability to recognise colours. Many of the activities focus on team games, something which is promoted in the Scottish curriculum framework document. The activities may not be appropriate for very young children who are not able to cope with the rules associated with group games.

All the games assume that the children can understand and put into practice the following:

❑ The ability to listen and follow instructions.

❑ Understanding of the concepts: sit/stand, stop/start.

❑ The ability to find four corners of a room.

Some of the activities also involve body actions and movements, for example, hopping, jumping or skipping. Physical

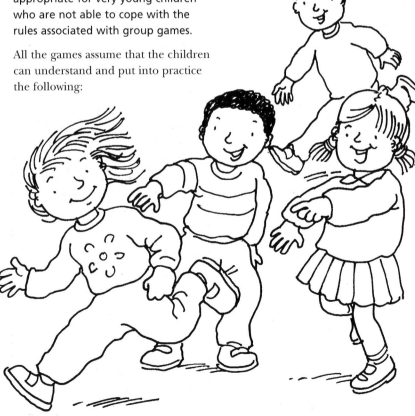

activities have to be based on realistic targets. In the suggested activities you should only be working on encouraging locomotion skills that you have previously been working on with the children. You will know what your children can do, so adapt these activities and choose physical skills appropriate to your group.
(See pages 9-10 for a list of types of physical skills).

Many of the suggested activities require the children to move quickly through space (ELG 4) and so a large working area is needed. Some of the activities could be carried out in smaller groups and may be more appropriate for the younger child or the child who is reluctant to work in a large space.

The activities may be more successful if there is more than one adult. However, as this is not always possible, introduce a few guidelines at the start of the session to make management of the group more effective. For example:

❑ When you put your hand up in the air the children have to stop what they are doing and sit down.

Noise levels may be higher than usual due to excitement or working in a larger space so always finish the session with a quieter activity.

To encourage the less able or less confident child make sure the groups have a mix of children.

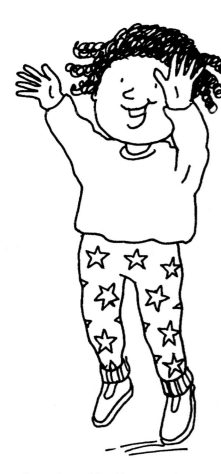

Learning objectives

The learning objectives are:

❏ To reinforce the children's knowledge of colours through physical activities.

❏ To listen and follow instructions.

❏ To move with confidence and control, show an awareness of space. (ELG 1, 4)

❏ To understand speed and be able to move safely. (ELG 1)

Ribbon games

Give the children coloured ribbons to wear. (Start with three or four colours, and increase the number of colours when they are able to cope with more.) Ask them to move round the room any way that they wish. When you call out their colour they have to freeze or sit down. Alter the game by asking them to hop or run round the room. You can make it more difficult by asking them, for example, to hop slowly round the room.

In smaller groups sit the children in a circle. When their colour is called, all the children wearing that colour ribbon have to run round the circle and back to their place. To extend the activity either change the way in which they have to move - hopping or skipping - or call out more than one colour!

Still wearing the coloured ribbons, the children move around the room, but this time when their colour is called they have to find a partner wearing the same colour ribbon as themselves.

Team games

These ideas are more appropriate for children working in the later stepping stones who are able to collaborate in devising and sharing tasks, including those which involve accepting rules. Place the children in teams standing at one end of the room. Have a selection of cards with a different colour on each card. At the other end of the room have a box full of coloured items which match the colour on the cards. Hold up one of the coloured cards. In their teams the children take it in turns to run to the box of items and find an object which matches the colour. Once they have found one they return with it to their team. Make it more difficult for older children by asking them to hop to the box or jump to the box.

Traffic lights

The children work individually for this game. You need three cards the colour of traffic lights. Red means stop, green means go and amber can mean slow down or quicken up. The children begin by standing still. Once the green card is held up they can move round the room. Alter their speed by showing the amber card and expect them to stop when you hold up the red card.

Colour corners

In each corner of the room place a coloured card. Begin with red, blue,

Other activities

❏ Making stained glass windows. (Creative Development)

❏ Using coloured playdough. (Physical Development/Creative development)

❏ Colour the water in the water tray. (Knowledge and Understanding of the World)

green and yellow; later they can be changed. Encourage the children to move round the room. When you shout out a colour, the children all have to run into the corresponding colour corner. Increase the level of difficulty in the way they are asked to move around.

Have the children sitting quietly in a space in the room or hall. Give them different coloured ribbons to wear. Begin to tell a story - it can be one you create as you go along. When you say their colour in the story they have to do an action of their choice. An alternative for older children is to have them sitting in two rows, facing each other with their legs stretched out in front of themselves. Each pair is given a colour. When they hear their colour in the story they stand up and run down between the two rows of children, over all the legs and back round to their place.

Books

Elmer's Colours David McKee (Anderson Press).

Maisie's Colours Lucy Cousins (Walker Books).

The Mixed up Chameleon Eric Carle (Picture Puffin).

Red, Yellow, Blue, Green (Images series Heinemann).

Planning for Learning through Colour Penny Coltman and Rachel Linfield (Step Forward Publishing).

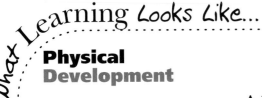

Physical Development

All about me

Look what I can do!

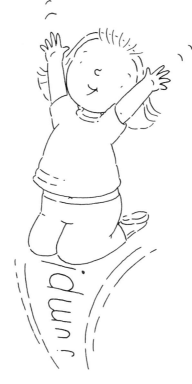

This is a vast theme, which could include all aspects of development. I have placed particular emphasis here on self-awareness, focusing on aspects of the child's physical and perceptual development. For example, asking questions such as 'What size are you?' and 'How do you move?'

Learning objectives

These activities are designed to help the children become more aware of what they can do with their bodies.

❑ Develop an awareness of specific body movements and move with confidence, imagination and in safety (ELG 1)

❑ Name body parts/body movements.

❑ Share and celebrate their achievements with their peer group.

❑ Use small equipment. (Stage 3)

Such a theme emphasises the similarities and differences between children. More importantly, perhaps, it fosters an understanding of their own needs and the needs of others.

This topic is a very personal one and the starting point, naturally, has to be with the child!

Simple games and songs

For younger children at stage 1 you could start by playing simple games, for example 'Simon says' or 'Follow my leader' - activities which are designed to encourage the children to use and name body parts. Most young children

will recognise the usual parts - hair, mouth, ears and nose - from a relatively young age. Introduce more difficult parts and see if they can find them, for example, wrists, neck, shoulder, chin, thigh or knuckle.

Singing songs such as 'I'm a dingly, dangly scarecrow' or 'I have a body, a very busy body' also reinforces their knowledge of body parts. Extend the activity further and move from body parts to body actions.

What can you do?

A simple question such as 'What can you do with your bodies?' can lead to a lively discussion. Children love showing others what they can do - the difficulty may be in having every child wanting to show you at the same time! Managing the group effectively will be something you decide as a team. I would ask them

to sit in a circle. Give each child in turn the opportunity to answer the question. The rest of the group can watch and then copy the answer.

Another way may be to listen to their answers, recording all their replies on a large piece of paper, which can be displayed in the classroom or the hall and added to as and when. Once you have a good range of answers, give the children the opportunity to use a larger space (ELG 4) and use the whole room or hall to try out some of the actions. They can all try out the same action together at first. Once they are confident in using the space and are beginning to control and co-ordinate their bodies more effectively (ELG 2) let them explore freely just what their bodies can do. Come together near the end of the session to give them time to share their findings with each other.

Big and small movements

For children at stage 2 the initial starting point may be the same - 'What can you do with your bodies?' - but may focus on gross motor and fine motor activities. Often when we talk about our bodies, we tend to focus only on large movements. Help the children to think about all the small movements we do - blinking our eyelids, wriggling our toes, bending our knees or clicking our fingers.

This may well be a quite open-ended movement session, concentrating on giving the children the opportunity to experiment, to practise and to discover just what their bodies can do. The

Welsh document stresses that by the time the children are five, their nursery experiences should enable them to understand, appreciate and enjoy the differences between actions. The document gives the examples of running, walking, skipping, jumping and hopping. This activity may well reinforce these differences.

Ask the children to classify body movements. For example:

❑ Body movements involving movement in space - tiptoing, walking, galloping and skipping.

❑ Body movements taking place at ground level - kneeling, swimming, crawling, curling and sliding.

❑ Body movements which are achieved when stationary - balancing, nodding their head, standing and blinking their eyes.

Can the children think of any more examples? Are they able to interchange the actions? Can they tiptoe when stationary? If not, why not?

Introducing small equipment

At stage 3, activities can be similar but also involve the use of small equipment. Asking them, 'What can you do with your bodies?' is the same, but the ideas and outcomes certainly won't be!

Using small apparatus or equipment (ELG 7) is important for a number of reasons. In addition to giving the children the opportunity to use their bodies in a different way, whilst having fun, using equipment also:

❑ Enhances co-ordinated movement (ELG 2)

❑ Develops balance (ELG 2)

❑ Stimulates the imagination (Scottish document)

❑ Encourages number, shape and colour work (Mathematics)

❑ Encourages the social skills of turn taking, sharing, co-operating and negotiating emphasised in the Scottish document.

The Scottish document also encourages staff to remember that children need to be helped to understand safe practices when using small apparatus and equipment. You may therefore want to proceed to stage 3 activities with some safe advice.

Try using the following:

Bean bags	Hoops
Quoits	Bells
Balloons	Ribbon
Tapsticks	Scarves
Tambourines	Balls
Short and long ropes	

Let the children choose one piece of equipment. Limit them to only one choice at this stage. If given the opportunity to have several different pieces of equipment in one session some children will spend the time choosing item after item rather than focusing on being creative. To spark off some ideas, ask the children first to use their chosen item to think of ways of making it move (not themselves at this point). Can they roll, tap, bounce, slide, balance, hit, throw, squeeze or throw their piece of equipment? Perhaps later the children can group the items under headings of what can/cannot be done with them.

Extend the activity and encourage the children to explore what they are able to do with the equipment (as above) and move at the same time. For example, bouncing a ball and walking, balancing a bean bag on their head and hopping or holding a balloon between their knees and sliding. The children will have more creative ideas!

Assessment

Assessing these activities may not only be difficult but may interrupt the children's creativity and imagination. It may be more appropriate to photograph the children in action. The photos can then be displayed with a selection of books on the theme. The children can make their own 'All by myself' books which can detail all the movements they can do unaided and is one way of celebrating success and recording achievement.

Other activities

❑ Making books - 'All by myself'. (Creative Development/ Communication, Language and Literacy)

❑ Record favourite body movements (hopping, running) on bar charts/pie charts. (Mathematical Development)

❑ Paint portrait pictures of themselves in action. (Creative Development)

❑ List similarities/differences between the children. (Knowledge and Understanding of the World)

Books and resources

Planning for Learning through All About Me Penny Coltman and Rachel Linfield (Step Forward Publishing).

All about Me Debbie MacKinnon/Anthea Sieveking (Francis Lincoln).

Look, See and Touch D Edwards (Methuen).

Who's that in the Mirror? P Berends (Random).

Physical
Development

People who help us

Stop, look, listen!

Through a theme on road safety and people who help us cross the road the children will be involved in developing a number of skills. They will learn how to collect data and interpret information. They will be discussing ideas and sharing personal information. They will be building up information on the local environment, as well as fulfilling some of the Early Learning Goals for Physical Development.

Learning objectives

The learning objectives for these activities are for the children:

❑ To use their bodies to stop, look and listen. (ELG for movement)

❑ To move in a controlled, co-ordinated and safe way when crossing the road.

❑ To understand speed and be able to stop/go when asked.

❑ To understand directional and positional words such as forwards, over, across, left and right.

At the same time, you can help children to recognise who they should ask to help them cross the road safely; recognise safe crossing places; and begin to understand the Green Cross Code.

Getting started

Ask the children how many of them walk to school or pre-school? Record the information on a simple bar graph - those who walk and those who do not. Which group has the most children? Ask the children who do not walk to school, why they don't. Could they

perhaps walk one day a week? (This is a good opportunity to promote ELG 5 - recognising the importance of keeping healthy and those things which contribute to this.) For children at stages 2 and 3 you may widen the discussion and list all the different ways of getting to school. Once they have done this, can they give each one a 'health' rating? (walking or cycling has a higher rating than coming by car)

Do they have to cross the road? Who is there to help them? Talk about the lollipop lady or man. (If there isn't a school crossing patrol nearby you will need to explain what a lollipop person does, perhaps show some pictures or even invite one in to talk to the children and show them their 'lollipop'.)

Together build up a profile on this person. What is their name? What is their job? What sort of clothing do they wear and why? Why is their job so important and in what way do they help us? Children at stage 1 could paint or draw pictures of this person. Children at stages 2 and 3 could write about them or create books displaying the information they have collected.

Stop

This activity can be done in a large group. The children have to be able to listen and follow instructions. You need to be in a large space - indoors or outdoors. Start by drawing their attention to the importance of speed and the speed of reactions. At all stages, begin by asking the children to move round the space. (ELG 4) At first they should just walk. When you shout

'Stop!' they have to stop. Even children working within the earliest stepping stones for movement should have the ability to stop. (You could also use a simplified version of the traffic lights game explained on page 53 - when you hold up a red circle they stop, a green circle means go.) Repeat the game but this time they have to jog and later run round the space. At what speed was it easier to stop? Why?

For children at stages 2 and 3 introduce a short racecourse. As children move through the stepping stones, they will have the ability to adjust speed or change direction to avoid obstacles. In turn the children can be asked to walk, jog or run. One child races whilst the other children stand at regular intervals along the side of the course - they are the markers. The child who is racing is asked to stop opposite one of the markers. How far further on from the marker has the child run before stopping? Explain that this is called the stopping distance. Measure this distance. When all the children have had a go, work out which child had the best stopping reaction. Again discuss whether it's easier to stop when walking, jogging or running. Comment on their findings and the implications they have for people crossing roads and for drivers. What other factors may contribute to a slower or faster stopping reaction? What does the lollipop lady do to stop the traffic? Children at stage 3 could design and make their own lollipop.

Look

These activities will be more successful if they are done with small groups.

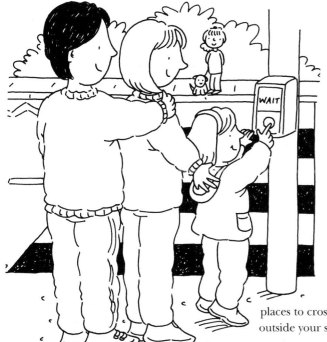

They involve going outside and so will also be safer in small groups with a good adult:child ratio. The children who stay behind can be engaged in a variety of activities related to the theme.

Use the opportunity to focus on looking by going outside and watching the traffic. For children at stage 1 compile a simple road traffic survey. Before going outside, draw up a list of all the vehicles the children can think of which use the roads. Together choose four or five vehicles. Produce a simple chart with pictures of the chosen vehicles. Outside encourage the children to make a mark each time they see the appropriate vehicle. Which vehicle did they see the most/least of?

Children at stage 2 may do a similar activity, but you can encourage them to look at the traffic and estimate how fast/slow the vehicles are moving - how did they decide on the speed? Why do we have different speeds on different types of road? Can they find out the speed limit for the road outside school? Another person who helps us is the policeman/woman (perhaps they can be invited in to talk about road safety). They may be able to show the children the equipment they use to track how fast a vehicle is travelling.

At stage 3 encourage the children to think about where is a safe place to cross a road. (Encourage them also to think of the places where it would be unsafe to cross, for example, on a bend

or between parked cars.) Once they have found a safe place, what do they have to look for before crossing the road? Extend this work by asking them to draw and sequence the Green Cross Code or draw and write about safe places to cross a road, particularly outside your setting.

Listen

These activities take place both inside and out. Again, it may be more appropriate to have a small group of children. For the indoor activities, if possible, use a quiet room or corner where the children cannot be distracted.

In our noisy world, children often hear sounds but do not really listen. Before taking them outside have small groups of children in a quiet corner. (The activity is the same for all stages; however, children at stage 3 can be given more sounds to listen to and more obscure ones, too.)

Begin by asking the children to think of as many vehicles as they can. Ask them what noise each vehicle makes - often children have quite simple sounds for each vehicle, and ones that sound nothing like the actual sound! Introduce a vehicle sound lotto. (Most educational suppliers sell these.) How many vehicles can the children identify? Are there any that they are unfamiliar with? (This activity can later be played independently using headsets if necessary.) Once they are familiar with the vehicle sounds, take them outside. Encourage them to keep very still and listen to all the sounds they can hear. When you feel they are ready, have some of the children facing the road, the others with their backs to the road. How good are the children with their backs to the road at identifying individual vehicles? Get the children facing the road to check if

they are correct/incorrect. Were there any vehicles they heard which they could not identify or which they had not heard on the tape?

If it is appropriate, involve your local Road Safety Officer and bring the 'stop, look and listen' activities together. The Road Safety Officer should be able to provide a range of resources to use with children of all ages. Children at all stages, though, will enjoy imaginative or role play. Ask the officer if they can bring along some examples of street furniture - zebra crossings, traffic lights, pelican crossings and clothes for policemen/women or lollipop men/women - for the children to create a road layout. Some of the children can pretend to be vehicles (or use ride-on toys), whilst other children are the 'people who help us' or pedestrians. Can the cars move safely, stopping when necessary? Can the pedestrians cross the road safely? For children who are able, this is also a good activity for encouraging their understanding of left and right.

Reinforce the message that even when there is someone there to help them cross the road they should never just step out onto the road before stopping, looking and listening. We have to give vehicles the chance to see us, slow down and stop in time.

Books and addresses

Crossing Roads Althea and L Newsham (Dinosaur).

The Hedgehog Dick King-Smith (Hamish Hamilton).

Sue Learns to Cross the Road Nigel Snell (Hamish Hamilton).

RoSPA has a wide variety of road safety materials. For a Safety Education Resources Catalogue, phone 0121 248 2000.

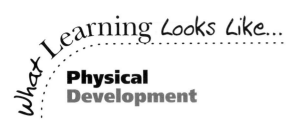

Physical Development

Planning for Physical Development

These pages show you how the 15 activities in the book cover all the ELGs for Physical Development.

There is much overlap between the goals. I have tried to place each activity under one ELG. However, most activities fulfil more than one goal.

For example:

❑ Moving with confidence, imagination and in safety. (ELG 1)

❑ Moving with control and co-ordination. (ELG 2)

❑ Showing awareness of space, of themselves and of others. (ELG 4)

are all very much interrelated. This is because if you are able to succeed in one of these goals you have probably also mastered the skills of the other two goals.

Having the ability to travel around, under, over and through balancing and climbing equipment is one goal which is difficult to cover through the themed activities. With very young children you should never be tempted to introduce large apparatus too soon. At this age it is best to concentrate on the earlier goals, encouraging them to develop their skills of control and co-ordination and awareness of space. It may be enough to be using outdoor play equipment, such as the climbing frame, to develop this goal.

Similarly many activities involve hand and finger skills and so will fulfil the goal of handling tools and objects.

Move with confidence, imagination and in safety (ELG 1)

Using a parachute

I can be a car!

Movement patterns

People who help us: Stop, look, listen

All about me: Look what I can do!

Water: Noah's ark

Move with control and co-ordination (ELG 2)

Using a parachute

I can be a car!

Movement patterns

All about me: Look what I can do!

Water: Noah's ark

Colour: Ribbon games and traffic lights

Travel around, under, over and through balancing and climbing equipment (ELG 3)

Using a parachute

I can be a car!

Show awareness of space, of themselves and of others (ELG 4)

I can be a car!

Movement patterns

All about me: Look what I can do!

Water: Noah's ark

People who help us: Stop, look, listen

Recognise the importance of keeping healthy and those things which contribute to this (ELG 5)

Healthy eating: The Very Hungry Caterpillar

Keeping healthy

Colour: Ribbon games and traffic lights

Recognise the changes that happen to their bodies when they are active (ELG 6)

How our bodies work

Keeping healthy

Use a range of small and large equipment (ELG 7)

I can be a car!

Movement patterns

Developing ball skills

All about me: Look what I can do!

Water: Noah's ark

Seasons: Sorting seeds

Handle tools, objects, construction materials safely and with increasing control (ELG 8)

Handling construction materials

Using a parachute

Wrapping presents and parcels

Seasons: Sorting seeds

Playing with dough

Developing ball skills

	ELG 1	ELG 2	ELG 3	ELG 4	ELG 5	ELG 6	ELG 7	ELG 8
Playing with dough	■							■
Movement patterns	■	■				■	■	
I can be a car!	■	■						
Wrapping presents and parcels								■
Handling construction materials		■						■
Using a parachute								■
Developing ball skills							■	
Healthy eating					■			
How our bodies work					■	■		
Keeping healthy					■			
Seasons: Sorting seeds	■			■				■
Water: Noah's ark		■		■				
Colour: Ribbon games and traffic lights	■	■						
All about me: Look what I can do!	■			■				
People who help us: Stop, look, listen								